NOVEL CORONAVIRUS:

GUIDE

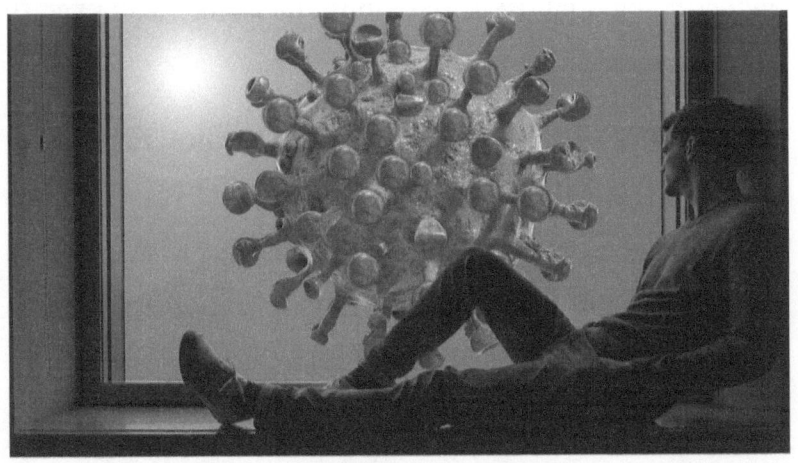

Dr. Mario Vega Carbó

Endocrinologist

Edition 2021

-Volume N° 1-

The author

Mario Vega Carbó he is a Cuban doctor, specialized in endocrinology, nutrition and family medicine, with over 20 years of experience.

He graduated in 1994 at the Institute of Medical Sciences of Havana (ISCMH) and then continued his training, completing a Master in Satisfactory Longevity, a specialization in Diagnostic Ultrasound and several courses in Higher Medical Education and Endocrinology.

His career began at the La Lisa Municipal Health Directorate and continued at the National Institute of Endocrinology and at the Polyclinic on July 26 in Cuba. Since 2014, he has worked as an endocrinologist at the Vega & Vado Clinic in Managua, Nicaragua.

Mario is also a professor of medical pathophysiology and likes to do good, family and nature.

He previously published *"Answering 1,500 questions about hormones, metabolism and nutrition"*, where he explains the causes of the main endocrine diseases, their most common symptoms, their risks and the best way to treat them.

Also *"Revealing Myths: Metabolism, Endocrinology and Reproduction"*, which tells the truth about popular beliefs related to diet, obesity, diabetes, cholesterol, hypertension, hair loss, puberty, infertility, sexuality and contraceptives.

"Novel-coronavirus guide" volume 1, is another of the texts aimed at understanding the general public is his third book.

Social Network:

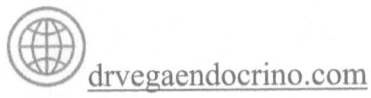 drvegaendocrino.com

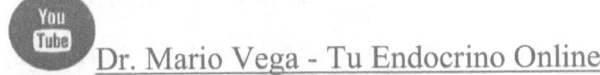 Dr. Mario Vega - Tu Endocrino Online

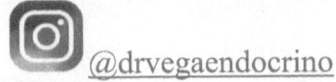 @drvegaendocrino

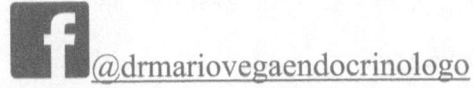 @drmariovegaendocrinologo

To the planet earth, the only one favored in this pandemic.

The glory of the Lord for each deceased,

and my condolences to their families and friends.

An appeal to the common sense of the entire human race.

My infinite love to my family and my friends.

My highest respects to my colleagues and to all health workers.

Volume 1

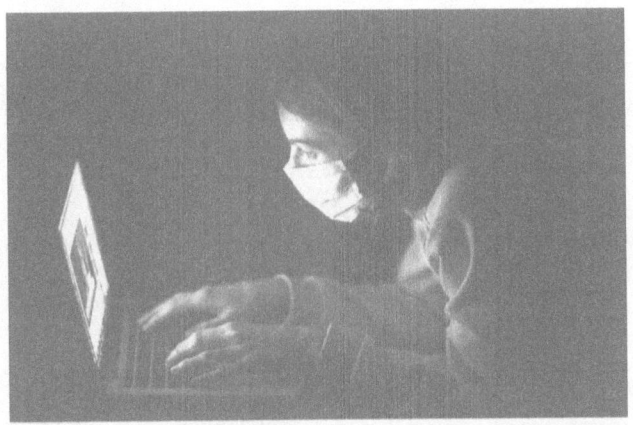

Aimed at the general public, to help you better understand the novel-coronavirus and its disease.

Introduction to Volume 1

Coronavirus and pandemics in the age of globalization

We live in a time that will be written in history. Until a few months ago, hardly anyone had heard about the coronavirus and COVID-19. However, today this disease is on everyone's lips and its impacts plunged the world into an unprecedented global and social crisis.

In addition to the worrying health issue, forced paralysis in activities is seriously affecting the economies of most countries, causing recession, isolation and uncertainty.

But, *how is it possible that a virus that emerged in China puts humanity's health and productive development at risk?*

Globalization and the constant movement of people make us all exposed to the latent threat of a pandemic.

Since the beginning of the 21st century, other contagious viral diseases, such as influenza, Middle East respiratory syndrome (MERS), SARS and the Ebola virus, have foretold the possibility of such a crisis.

In a short time, the new coronavirus spread throughout the world and the severity of the situation is forcing extreme measures to be taken to try to stop them from spreading.

Just like the black plague or smallpox in their time, this disease poses a challenge that implies new challenges and requires novel solutions to overcome it.

As there is no specific cure so far, the best way to deal with it is through knowledge, research and the dissemination of proven techniques to control and prevent it.

Within this framework, Dr. Mario Vega Carbó presents a new book on COVID-19, with the aim of offering information to the population in general and to health practitioners in particular.

In a simple language to which we are accustomed, this specialist enters fully into the world of viral diseases, making available to everyone a manual that serves as a guide to better understand the new coronavirus, its effects and consequences.

It analyzes its history and characteristics, the way it is transmitted, its most common symptoms and the complications it generates in the human body.

It also explores the groups at greatest risk and the prevention and protection measures that must be taken at the personal, local, national and international levels to prevent their spread.

It also evaluates the types of treatments available and the way in which patients affected by the disease must be cared for and managed.

As an introduction, Dr. Mario answers the basic questions about this virus:

-Doctor, what specifically is the new coronavirus?

It is the causative agent of a new disease, officially named COVID-19 by the World Health Organization (WHO), it is a respiratory disease similar to the flu, but highly contagious.

Its causative agent belongs to the family of coronaviruses, which are a series of viruses that cause everything from a common cold to more serious conditions, such as Middle East respiratory syndrome (MERS-CoV) and severe acute respiratory syndrome (SARS-CoV).

-What are your most common symptoms?

Its most common clinical signs are cough, sore throat and headache, runny nose, shortness of breath, tiredness and fever.

Most people take 2 to 14 days to show symptoms after being infected, and these signs generally last for a week and after which there is usually improvement.

However, in people with a weak immune system, or with various underlying diseases, such as in the elderly, the condition can be more serious and cause pneumonia, bronchitis, kidney failure, heart damage, and even death, so it is essential to take all kinds of care.

-How is this disease spread?

COVID-19 disease is spread through direct contact or with secretions from infected people, such as saliva drops expelled with a cough or sneeze.

Also by touching an object or surface that has the virus and then passing your hands through your mouth, eyes or nose before washing them properly.

-How is this ailment diagnosed?

To confirm this disease, special laboratory tests of respiratory or blood samples are needed.

They study the genetic markers of the virus to identify it and rule out other ailments.

-How is COVID-19 treated?

At the moment there is no specific treatment for this disease, but doctors can prescribe medications for pain or fever.

In most cases, people recover by resting and drinking plenty of fluids, and symptoms clear up on their own within a few days.

When the patient has difficulty breathing, is unable to retain fluids, or suffers from other pre-existing conditions, it is important that a doctor be contacted immediately to see the next steps.

The same for those belonging to risk groups, such as the elderly, pregnant women or those with compromised immune systems.

-How can we prevent its spread?

To prevent transmission of COVID-19, it is recommended to wash your hands frequently, especially before eating and after using the bathroom, blowing your nose, coughing, or sneezing.

If you can't do it, you can use an alcohol-based hand sanitizer with at least 60% of this compound.

You should also avoid touching your eyes, nose and mouth; and disinfect everyday objects and surfaces with cleaning sprays.

The use of face masks or face masks is advisable, not so much as a general measure, but if for those who have the disease and prevent it from spreading, or for those who are health professionals.

When coughing or sneezing, cover yourself with a handkerchief or the elbow sleeves, avoiding using your hands.

On the other hand, you can get a flu shot if you haven't received it this season yet.

Remember that with more information we can take better care of each other and reduce transmission risks.

I invite you to read this manual to know everything you need about COVID-19 and contagious viral diseases.

Part I. Defenses, airways and viruses

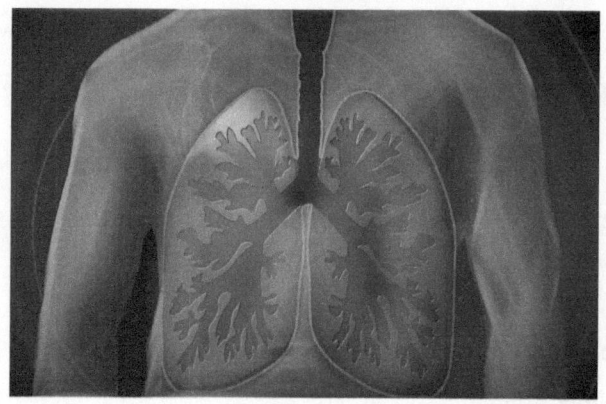

1. Types of Immunity. Examples

-Doctor Mario, what is the immune system?

The immune system is the body's natural defense against infection and germs.

It is made up of cells, tissues and organs that work together to detect, fight and destroy certain pathogens before they cause damage to the body.

-How does this system work?

To prevent the entry of germs, the body has external barriers such as the skin and mucosa. When these are overcome, pathogens enter the body and begin to damage it.

To combat this attack, the immune system has a first line of defense formed by leukocytes or white blood cells. These cells are found in the blood and can be moved to various places in the body to protect it.

Once they detect the entry of microorganisms or foreign substances, the leukocytes penetrate the tissues and, upon contact with the invaders, generate antibodies to destroy them.

- What does the concept of immunity refer to?

Immunity is a state of natural or acquired resistance that some individuals or species possess against the attack of an infectious or toxic agent.

In medicine, this concept refers to the protection that the immune system offers the body against diseases.

-How many types of immunity are there?

There are two types: the innate and the acquired. The first is an immunity that is available by inheritance or by biological means. Some individuals or species have the characteristic of not suffering or transmitting certain diseases, even if they have never been in contact with the agent that causes them.

Innate immunity also refers to the defense system you are born with.

Acquired, on the other hand, is a type of immunity that is achieved after exposure to a certain pathogen. In these cases the body generates antibodies and then "remembers" the invader and builds a specific defense to prevent a similar new infection in the future.

-Could you give us examples of each type of immunity?

The cough reflex, gastric acid, mucus, and tears are examples of innate immunity.

Meanwhile, the protection obtained from vaccines is a case of acquired immunity.

2. Humoral and cellular immunity

What is humoral immunity?

It is a type of acquired immunity in which the immune system recognizes potentially dangerous invading agents and produces antibodies to destroy them.

When the threat is eliminated, cells store this information in memory so that they can respond more quickly to future attacks by the same germ.

-What is cellular immunity?

It is another type of acquired immunity in which, against an invading agent, the cells of the immune system release specific substances called cytokines to destroy them, without the intervention of antibodies.

-What is the difference between both types?

Broadly speaking, we can say that humoral immunity acts against extracellular microorganisms and cellular immunity against intracellular microorganisms.

In the first, the attack occurs with antibodies that inactivate or mark potentially dangerous agents to be destroyed, while in the second they are directly attacked by cells.

3. Active and passive immunity

-What is active immunity?

It is a type of acquired immunity in which our own body generates specific antibodies against a certain pathogen after having suffered from it.

An example of this is vaccines, in which attenuated viruses are administered to the body so that the body produces durable and resistant defenses against it.

-What is passive immunity?

It is a type of acquired immunity in which the antibodies against a certain invader are produced by a different organism than the person.

For example, these are the defenses that are passed from mother to child through milk or the placenta, or when blood serum from an immune donor is supplied to a sick patient.

4. Defense against biological agents

-What are biological agents?

Biological agents are all those microorganisms which can cause any type of infection, allergy or toxicity to humans.

These can have different shapes and sizes. The best known are viruses, bacteria, fungi, human endoparasites (protozoa and helminths) and prions.

-What are viruses?

Viruses are organisms with a very simple structure, they can reproduce themselves within certain cells, using their metabolism.

They are very small germs that invade living cells and use them to multiply, causing them to become damaged, mutate, die, or become sick.

These organisms are responsible for producing infectious ailments such as the cold, flu, AIDS, smallpox, measles, and COVID-19.

-How is the defense against these biological agents?

When an attack occurs, the body first tries to prevent these invaders from entering. If these manage to enter, the immune system looks for a way to fight and destroy them.

In the event that these actions are not entirely effective, pathogens settle in the body and cause diseases.

5. Anatomy of the airways

-What are the airways?

The airways are the set of organs that make breathing possible.

The cells of our body need oxygen to live. Through respiration, oxygen enters our body and allows the carbon dioxide generated by cells to exit when they do their job.

-What organs are part of the airways?

The respiratory system is made up of the nose, pharynx, larynx, trachea, bronchi, bronchioles, and lungs.

In addition, different structures, such as the diaphragm and intercostal muscles, also participate in breathing.

-What happens to the oxygen once it enters our body?

When it enters our body, it is inhaled into the lungs and passes through the thin membranes of the alveoli into the bloodstream.

There, hemoglobin captures it in red blood cells and flows to the heart, which pumps this oxygen-rich blood to the tissues of the body that need it, through the arteries.

6. Barriers, mucosa and respiratory epithelium

-How do germs enter our body through the respiratory tract?

When we breathe the air that enters our body is not completely clean. It contains chemicals and organic particles such as dust, bacteria, fungi, viruses and pollen that can be harmful to our health.

-What are the defense mechanisms of the respiratory system?

The respiratory system has a series of physical barriers to prevent the entry of germs. These include nasal hairs, mucosa, cough, and sneezing.

When these defenses fail to prevent the entry and development of pathogens, the immune system itself becomes operational.

-What are mucous membranes?

The mucous membranes are a series of membranes that surround the entire respiratory system, from the larynx to the bronchi, to protect it. For this, they secrete a dense and sticky substance that covers the internal walls of these organs.

When harmful agents enter the body through the airways and overcome nasal hair, they are attracted to this slimy mucus, where they become trapped and are then expelled through the nose and mouth.

-What happens when we sneeze or cough?

When too large particles enter the body to be trapped by the sticky substance of the mucosa, the body activates emergency mechanisms to try to expel them.

In the case of sneezing and coughing, there is a stimulation of nerve receptors, which remove a large amount of air from the body at high speed, seeking to also drag a foreign body.

-What is the respiratory epithelium?

This epithelium is a tissue that covers the surface, cavities, and ducts of the respiratory tract, moistening and protecting it. It works as a barrier against foreign particles and pathogens, preventing infections and damage.

7. Acute respiratory infections

-What are acute respiratory infections?

They are respiratory tract infections with evolution less than 15 days that can be transmitted from person to person.

They can be mild, moderate or severe and constitute a major cause of death worldwide, mainly in children under 5 years of age and adults over 65 years of age.

-What are the most common symptoms of an acute respiratory infection?

Its most frequent signs include fever, cough, lethargy, and difficulty breathing. Also sore throats, headaches, chest and joint pain.

-What is the main complication that these infections can cause?

In severe cases these infections can generate pneumonia, where a certain virus or bacteria causes inflammation of the lungs. This disease is characterized by symptoms such as high fever, chills, severe pain in the chest, cough and secretions, and can be fatal.

8. Most common respiratory viruses

-What are the most common respiratory viruses?

The most frequent viruses are the Respiratory Syncytial Virus, the Rhinovirus, the influenza and the adenoviruses.

-What is the Respiratory Syncytial Virus?

It is a virus that causes lung and respiratory tract infections, mainly in babies, young children, and older adults.

Its symptoms vary depending on the age of the infected. They are generally moderate and include cough, nasal congestion, and low fever.

In more severe cases there may be difficulty breathing and blue discoloration as a result of lack of oxygen.

-What is rhinovirus?

It is a virus that can cause a common cold, pharyngitis, ear infections, and sinusitis. In a few cases, it can also cause pneumonia and bronchiolitis.

Rhinovirus is one of the most common human pathogens and is easily spread from person to person.

-What is influenza?

It is the influenza virus, which mainly attacks the nose, throat and lungs. It is easily contagious and has an incubation period of between 1 and 3 days.

Its symptoms are similar to those of a cold, although a little more sudden and sudden. These include a runny nose, sneezing, and a sore throat.

This virus usually goes away on its own, but in some cases it can lead to more serious complications.

-What are adenoviruses?

They are a type of virus that, in addition to the airways, can infect the membranes of the eyes, intestines, urinary tract, and nervous system.

They cause fever, colds, conjunctivitis, diarrhea, bronchitis and pneumonia, among other ailments.

Adenoviruses attack people of any age, although they are more frequent in children.

9. Bacterial over-infections

-What are bacteria?

Bacteria are single-celled microorganisms that proliferate in different types of environments. Most of them are not harmful and some are even essential for the human body, such as those involved in the digestion of food.

However, about 1% can be harmful to health and cause disease.

-How are they different from viruses?

Viruses are smaller and need live hosts to survive, since they have no mechanisms of their own. Bacteria, on the other hand, have the property to grow and reproduce on their own.

However, from a medical point of view the main difference is that antibiotics often kill bacteria but are ineffective against viruses.

-What is bacterial superinfection?

It is a concept that is used in medicine for cases of a viral respiratory infection to which a bacterial complication is added.

When this occurs, the bacteria make it easier for the virus to replicate and vice versa, which makes the infection worse, and can even be fatal.

10. Upper and lower respiratory complications

-How are respiratory infections classified?

They are classified as high and low, depending on which is the affected area.

The high ones afflict from the nostrils to the vocal cords in the larynx, passing through the paranasal sinuses and the middle ear.

Low respiratory infections, in turn, include those that afflict from the trachea and bronchi to the bronchioles and alveoli.

-What are the most common upper respiratory complications?

The most common are rhinitis (common cold), sinusitis, influenza, ear infections, tonsillitis, pharyngitis and laryngitis. The vast majority of these infections are mild and have a natural beginning and end after a certain period of time.

-What are the most common complications of the lower respiratory tract?

In this case, the most common are bronchiolitis, influenza and pneumonia. In general, lower respiratory tract infections are usually more severe than upper respiratory infections.

Part II Virology, Coronavirus and COVID-19

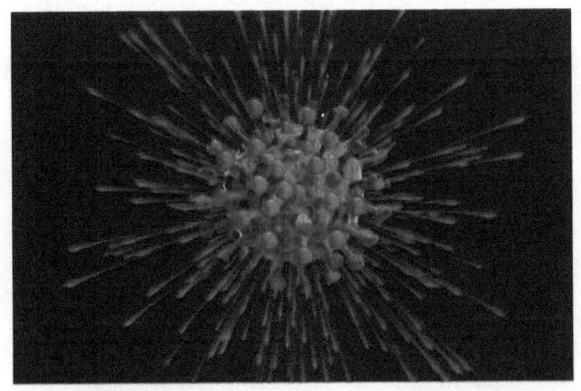

11. Types and characteristics of non-respiratory viruses

-*Doctor Mario, how are viral infections classified?*

These infections are classified according to the organ most affected by the virus. For example, in addition to respiratory infections, there are viral gastrointestinal, hepatic, neurological, and skin infections, among other types.

-*What can you tell us about gastrointestinal viral infections?*

Viral gastroenteritis is usually spread through contact with infected people or by eating contaminated food or liquids. Its most frequent signs are diarrhea, stomach cramps, vomiting and fever.

Among these viruses, rotavirus usually affects children; norovirus to older children and adults; and astrovirus and adenovirus in infants and young children.

-*And viral liver infections?*

Among these diseases is hepatitis. A is transmitted via the fecal-oral route; B through different body fluids such as blood, semen, and saliva; and C sexually or through blood.

In addition, other viruses that can affect the liver are cytomegalovirus, Epstein-Barr, yellow fever, and rubella.

-How are viral neurological infections?

These are a variable group of infections that affect the central nervous system and their causes can be infectious agents of various viral groups, as well as bacteria and also fungi.

Within viruses, there is a group called arboviruses, since they are generally transmitted to humans through the bite of arthropods that ingest blood, such as mosquitoes and ticks. Most cases of encephalitis, which involves inflammation of the brain due to infection, are viral.

-What other types of non-respiratory viruses are more recognized?

Among others we can mention herpesviruses, which cause mononucleosis, cold and genital herpes and chicken pox, among other diseases.

Also to the human papilloma virus, which causes epithelial lesions such as warts.

Other cases are the measles and mumps viruses, and HIV, which is transmitted sexually, by blood or breast milk, and causes AIDS.

12. Flu and viruses more aggressive to the respiratory tree

-*What is the flu and what causes it?*

The flu is a viral respiratory infection that infects the nose, throat and lungs. It is caused by the influenza virus that is spread from person to person and spreads easily.

When a patient coughs, sneezes, or talks, he expels small drops of air that can fall into the mouth or nose of people who are nearby.

In addition it is also possible to get infected by touching an object or surface that has the virus and then pass this hand through the mouth, nose or eyes.

-*What complications can the flu bring?*

In severe cases it can lead to pneumonia (inflammation of the lungs), encephalitis (inflammation of the brain), myocarditis (inflammation of the heart), meningitis (inflammation of the meninges), and seizures.

-What are the most aggressive respiratory viruses?

In addition to influenza, we can mention Marburg hemorrhagic fever, Ebola virus, hantavirus, avian influenza, swine influenza (H1N1) and coronaviruses.

-What is Marburg hemorrhagic fever?

It is a disease caused by one of the deadliest viruses, with a 90% mortality rate. It causes severe fever, headache, seizures, and bleeding from the mucosa, skin, and internal organs. At the moment there are no vaccines to combat it.

-What is the Ebola Virus?

It is a virus similar to the previous one, which causes hemorrhages throughout the body, fever and diarrhea. Its mortality rate is 70% and to date there are no vaccines either.

-What is hantavirus?

It is a group of viruses that are spread by exposure to the droppings of infected rodents. They cause fever and lung and kidney failure.

-What is bird flu?

It is a type of influenza that mainly affects birds, but can also be spread to humans. Its most common symptoms are high fever, diarrhea, vomiting, abdominal pain, and bleeding. Its mortality rate is 70%.

-What is swine influenza (H1N1)?

It is a type of flu transmitted by pigs. Its most common signs are fever, headache, cough, nausea, and vomiting.

13. Coronavirus: types, their shape and structure

-What are coronaviruses?

Coronaviruses are a broad family of viruses that can cause a variety of conditions, from a common cold to more serious illnesses, such as Middle East respiratory syndrome (MERS-CoV) and severe acute respiratory syndrome (SARS-CoV).

SARS-CoV-2, which causes COVID-19 disease, is a new strain that has not been found before in humans.

-How many types of coronaviruses are there?

There are a large number of coronaviruses that cause respiratory, gastrointestinal, liver, and neurological ailments in animals.

Of these, there are currently only 7 that can cause disease in humans. They are called HCovs (Human coronavirus).

-What is the shape and structure of coronaviruses?

This family of viruses is called coronaviruses because viewed under a microscope their surfaces have crown-shaped tips.

Its structure is made up of an envelope that contains a single chain of ribonucleic acid (RNA, the genetic material of the virus), and a glycoprotein lipid membrane from which several proteins with different functions protrude.

Among them, protein S enables the virus to enter cells, protein E is essential to infect others, and protein N allows them to hide genetic material.

14. Classification of coronaviruses

-What are the seven coronaviruses that affect humans?

The four most common are HCoV-229E, HCoV-OC43, HCoV-NL63, and HCoV-HKU1. These are not dangerous and are mainly found in non-life threatening colds. Most people are believed to have developed defenses against them and are immunized.

Of the remaining three, the first to appear was severe acute respiratory syndrome (SARS-CoV). It arose in China in 2002 and caused 800 deaths, with a fatality of 9.6%.

The second was the Middle East respiratory syndrome (MERS-CoV), which erupted in 2012 and spread to 27 countries in Asia, Europe, Africa and North America. It was more lethal than the previous one (34.5%) and caused 850 deaths.

The third is the current SARS-CoV-2 coronavirus, which emerged in China in late 2019 and spread almost everywhere in the world. Its mortality rate is relatively low compared to the other two, between 3 and 4%, but being so massive the number of victims is much higher.

15. Animal-borne coronaviruses

-What are the animals that transmit coronaviruses?

There are many wild animals that carry pathogens and are possible transmitters of contagious diseases. Among those we know may be host to the coronavirus are bats, civets, badgers, bamboo rats, and wild camels.

-How are coronaviruses transmitted from animals to humans?

In general, this type of contagion occurs when humans invade the spaces where wild animals live and when they are hunted to eat or to be sold.

Certain animals are used to living with certain viruses. The problem occurs when man handles these animals and the virus mutates to lodge and survive in other species.

While the animal that caused the current coronavirus outbreak is still unconfirmed, theories point to bats. The transmission of these animals to humans could have occurred after the mutation through one or more intermediate hosts.

-Why do these outbreaks generally arise in the East?

One of the reasons is the large number of inhabitants that many of these countries have.

The rapid urbanization that these regions are having, where nearly 60% of the world population already lives, makes them invade spaces where wild animals live. This forces closer proximity to human and domestic animal populations, facilitating contagion.

On the other hand, the eating habits of these countries, which include bats and snakes among other wild animals, often generate this type of development, as has previously happened with avian and swine flu, and with coronaviruses.

-Can our pets transmit coronavirus?

So far there is no evidence that companion animals, such as dogs or cats, can transmit this type of virus.

16. Resistance in different environments

-How long can coronaviruses live in environments?

In general, this class of virus has the ability to survive several hours on smooth surfaces and, if the temperature and humidity are adequate, can even last for days.

However, it is possible to quickly leave them inactive by using common disinfectants or by exposing them to higher temperatures.

-When does the new coronavirus last in the air?

The new coronavirus is believed to be able to survive in the air for at least 30 minutes.

-What is your survival from the new coronavirus to other environments?

Although there is still no conclusive data, a study carried out in China indicates that the survival time of the new coronavirus at different environmental temperatures is as follows:

-Air at 10-15 ° C: 4 hours.

-Cough drops at 25 ° C: 24 hours.

-Hands at 20-30 ° C: less than 5 minutes.

-Clothes at 10-15 ° C: less than 8 hours.

-Wood at 10-15 ° C: 48 hours.

-Stainless steel at 10-15 ° C: 24 hours.

17. Differences between COVID-19 and previous coronaviruses

-Which are the differences between the new coronavirus and the previous ones?

As I already mentioned, while COVID-19 is less lethal, it is much more infectious, causing it to spread rapidly.

Regarding the incubation period (the time between infection and the appearance of the symptoms of the disease), that of the new virus is between 2 and 14 days, while that of SARS is between 2 and 7 days and the from MERS 6 days.

18. Virulence of SARS-CoV-2

-How contagious and virulent is the new coronavirus?

To measure its virulence, both infectivity and lethality must be considered. SARS-CoV-2 is highly infectious and its case fatality rate is between 3 and 4 percent. This means that it is almost twice as contagious as influenza and therefore its mortality, although lower than influenza, accumulates rapidly.

However, it is less lethal than previous coronaviruses: the case fatality rate for SARS is 9.6 percent and for MERS 34.5 percent.

-What is the difference between epidemic and pandemic?

An epidemic is called a disease that spreads for some time through a certain country, simultaneously attacking large numbers of people.

This becomes a pandemic when the disease spreads to many countries or attacks almost all individuals in a locality or region.

-Why did this virus become a pandemic?

Due to the antigenic mutations suffered by the virus, humans do not have immunity against this strain.

This, in addition to the fact that there is more than one transmission route, caused the COVID-19 to spread throughout almost the entire world, affecting a significant number of people.

19. Immunity to COVID-19

-Can humans develop immunity to the new coronavirus?

It is still too early to give an answer. At the moment, there are no determining scientific data on the duration of the protective immune antibodies generated in patients who had the disease and were cured.

However, these patients may be protected from future infections.

- These recovered people would be immune to the virus for their entire lives?

Protective antibodies are generally produced two weeks after an infection and can last for several weeks or even many years in the body, preventing reinfection.

For example, antibodies raised against measles provide a lifetime of immunity. Meanwhile, those created against coronaviruses that cause a common cold last between one and three years.

-How was the immunity in SARS and MERS cases?

Most people who became infected with SARS developed long-term immunity, ranging from eight to ten years. In the case of MERS it was much shorter. It is estimated that immunity against COVID-19 could be at least 1 or 2 years, although at the moment there are no concrete data in this regard.

-What benefits could get those that are immune to the virus?

Immune people may help care for the seriously ill until a vaccine is released. Furthermore, their antibodies could be supplied to patients in need using blood serum.

On the other hand, increased immunity is also the way in which the pandemic is defeated, since as there are fewer people to infect, the virus loses strength and even vulnerable audiences are less exposed to contagion.

Part III. Risks and transmission between humans

20. Epidemiological characteristics

-Doctor Mario, what are the epidemiological stages of COVID-19?

The new coronavirus went through four stages since its inception: first it started as a local outbreak, then it continued with a community transmission, and it continued with a generalized contagion, which turned first into an epidemic and finally into a pandemic.

-How was the development of these stages?

In the case of China, where the outbreak originated, the local stage occurred mainly in the Wuhan market, where seafood, octopus, snakes, bats and badgers, among other animals, were sold.

Then the community broadcast attacked the entire city of Wuhan, through direct person-to-person contact.

Finally, the diffusion continued rapidly throughout the country and then spread to the rest of the world.

-How was the transmission dynamics in the Chinese case?

In the initial stage, the average incubation period for the virus was 5.2 days. Meanwhile, the number of infected people doubled every 7.4 days and the time interval of transmission from one person to another was 7.5 days.

It is estimated that each patient infected between 2.2 and 3.8 people on average. Regarding the age of those affected, 87 percent were people between 30 and 79 years old.

Of the total cases, 81 percent were mild, 14 percent severe, and 5 percent critical.

-*What was the average time interval from disease onset to hospitalization?*

In mild cases the interval was 5.8 days.

In severe cases, the interval until hospitalization was 7 days and 8 days until diagnosis.

Finally, for mortality cases, the interval until diagnosis was 9 days and 9.5 days until death.

-*How long does the infection by this virus last?*

The duration of the disease varies from person to person. Mild symptoms in a healthy individual can go away on their own within a few days, usually about a week, as in the case of the flu.

Conversely, recovery for a patient with other health problems can take weeks and, in severe cases, be life-threatening.

21. Most common transmission routes

-How does COVID-19 spread?

This disease is spread through direct contact or with secretions from infected people, such as cough drops or a sneeze.

Also by touching an object or surface that has the virus and then passing your hands through your mouth, eyes or nose before washing them properly.

In any case, the ways of propagation are still being investigated.

-Can the disease be transmitted through the air?

Studies carried out to date indicate that this virus is transmitted mainly by contact with respiratory drops rather than through the air.

However, there are reports confirming that the spread of the virus in the air is more sustained than what was considered at the beginning of the pandemic.

-Is it possible to get this disease from contact with a person who has no symptoms?

As the inhalation of the drops expelled by someone when coughing or sneezing is the main source of infection, the risk of contracting the disease of someone who does not show signs is low.

However, many people with COVID-19 only show mild symptoms. In this way, it is possible to get the virus from someone who, for example, has only a mild cough and does not feel sick.

-Is it possible to spread this ailment by contact with the feces of a sick person?

Although the first investigations show that in some cases the virus can be present in the feces of infected people, the risk of contagion seems to be low.

However, however unlikely it is, it is recommended to wash your hands frequently after using the bathroom and before eating.

-Can the disease be transmitted from mother to child?

The first studies indicate that there is no vertical transmission before, during and after childbirth from infected mothers to offspring. In any case, the investigation continues.

-Is it safe to shake hands with an infected person?

No. Respiratory viruses can be spread by shaking hands and then touching your eyes, nose, and mouth.

The safest thing is to avoid physical contact when greeting each other or doing it with a gesture, a bow of the head or a bow.

-Does rubber gloves help prevent virus infection?

No. The fact of using them does not prevent contagion since if the person touches his face with the glove, the virus can be transmitted in the same way as with the hand.

-Can I get COVID-19 from a blood transfusion?

At the moment there is no evidence to indicate that this coronavirus can be transmitted through a blood transfusion.

22. Transmission by air drops

-How is the transmission by drops areas?

Drops are small, spheroidal particles that contain water, with a diameter greater than 5 microns. The respiratory ones are generated mainly when coughing, sneezing or speaking.

These drops are thrown one or two meters from the person who emits them and can infect a person who is nearby and inhales them.

Due to their size and weight, the droplets do not remain suspended in the air for long, and quickly fall to the ground.

-What other ailments are transmitted through respiratory drops?

In addition to COVID-19, other viruses that are transmitted in this way include influenza, the SARS coronavirus, adenovirus, rhinovirus, mycoplasma, group streptococcus, and meningococcus.

-In what other circumstances can respiratory drops be generated?

These drops can also be generated during invasive respiratory tract procedures, such as aspiration or bronchoscopy, tracheal intubation, lung resuscitation, and cough-stimulating movements, such as changes in position in bed or patting on the back.

-How is transmission by air?

This type of contagion is known as aerosol transmission. Aerosols are suspensions of small particles or droplets less than 5 microns in diameter that contain pathogens.

So far the World Health Organization has assured that there is insufficient evidence to suggest that COVID-19 is transmitted by air, except in certain medical contexts, such as when an infected patient is intubated.

However, some scientists maintain that there is preliminary evidence that this type of contagion could occur. Therefore, it is recommended to take precautions, such as increasing the ventilation of the rooms, to reduce the risks.

23. Transmission by indirect contact

-How is transmission by indirect contact?

This type of transmission occurs when the drops that contain the virus are deposited on the surface of an object, such as a mobile phone or when we pass a ladder.

If a person touches those objects and then passes his/her hands through his mouth, eyes or nose, he can become infected.

-How long does this virus survive on a surface?

At the moment it is not known for sure. In general, this class of virus has the ability to survive several hours on smooth surfaces and, if the temperature and humidity are adequate, can even last for days.

However, it is possible to quickly leave them inactive by using common disinfectants or by exposing them to higher temperatures.

-Is it safe to receive a package from an area where COVID-19 cases have been reported?

Yes. The probability of contracting the virus by contact with a package that has been handled, transported and exposed to different conditions and temperatures is very low.

-What protection measures can be taken to avoid this type of infection?

Frequent hand washing using soap and water or an alcohol-based disinfectant is essential. Avoid touching your eyes, nose and mouth as well.

On the other hand, it is also important to disinfect objects and surfaces of daily use with cleaning sprays.

24. Risks for closer contacts

-What is meant by close contact?

Close contacts are all those who have a relationship with an infected or suspected patient.

This includes for example everyone who lives, studies or works with that person and also those who shared the same transport or elevator.

-What happens in the case of a patient who is hospitalized?

In this case, close contacts with doctors, hospital personnel, family or friends who have been with the patient without taking effective protection measures during their stay in the medical center are considered.

Also to other patients and their companions who share the same room with the infected.

25. Medical observation of contacts for 14 days

-Why should close contacts undergo a 14-day quarantine?

The incubation period (the time between infection and the appearance of disease symptoms) of the new virus is between 2 and 14 days.

Therefore, it is important to protect and monitor close contacts to detect if they are infected and at the same time prevent them from transmitting the disease to more people.

-What is avoided with this measure?

These people can be symptom-free for several days after becoming infected. This means that they appear completely healthy but are unknowingly transmitting the disease to others.

With quarantine this possible contagion is avoided. Therefore, it is important that people do not wait for signs of the disease to appear to isolate themselves.

26. Cutting the transmission chain

-*What is social distancing?*

Social distancing is a measure that public health officials recommend to decrease the spread of a disease that is transmitted from person to person.

When those infected by the virus stay away from others, they cannot infect anyone. In this way there are fewer sick people at the same time.

-*What is social distancing for?*

This measure serves to reduce the potential for disease transmission. If done correctly and on a large scale, social distance breaks or decreases the chain of contagion.

This helps protect vulnerable audiences and reduces the burden of care in hospitals, avoiding the collapse of the health system.

-What does social distancing imply?

This concept implies leaving a distance of more than two meters with other people; and avoid crowds, mass gatherings, and family and friend gatherings indoors.

Also avoid shaking hands, hugging or kissing other people; and not visiting vulnerable people, such as those in nursing homes or hospitals, babies, or people with compromised immune systems.

In irrigated areas everyone should stay at home as much as possible to avoid the spread of the virus.

-What massive measures are being taken in the affected communities to facilitate social distancing?

General quarantines are being decreed in many of the affected or at-risk communities. This includes the closure of non-essential factories, offices, banks, schools, theaters, cinemas, shopping malls, restaurants, gyms and shops, and the suspension of shows, sporting, cultural and social events.

Some countries have also closed their borders and are prohibiting citizens from going outside without justification.

27. Risk groups more susceptible to contagion

-Are there people who are more at risk of getting it than others?

Being a new strain of virus that has not been found before in humans, we are all susceptible to it for not having immunity.

If exposed to the virus, anyone can become infected, whether they have normal immune function or not.

For example, children are as much at risk of contracting the disease as adults. However, in general the symptoms in them are milder than in older people.

-Are there people who present more risks if they are infected?

Yes. People over the age of 60, those with respiratory or cardiovascular diseases, and those with conditions such as diabetes are at higher risk for infection.

Also, in those with poor immune function, such as the elderly, pregnant women, or people with liver or kidney dysfunction, the disease progresses relatively quickly and symptoms are more severe.

Part IV Cases, clinic and possible complications

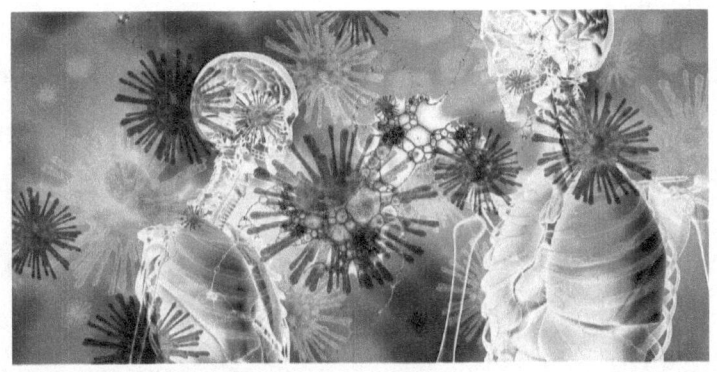

28. Subclinical cases

-Doctor Mario, what are the clinical manifestations of COVID-19?

In general, the first thing that appears in these patients is fever, although some only have chills and respiratory symptoms.

This may be accompanied by shortness of breath, dry cough, tiredness, and diarrhea, among other symptoms. Meanwhile, runny nose and phlegm are rare.

On the other hand, chest radiographs show characteristics of viral pneumonia and during the initial stage of the disease the white blood cell count is normal or lower than normal, while the lymphocyte count may decrease.

-In what percentages do these symptoms occur at the beginning of the infection?

Fever appears in 88% of cases. While dry cough occurs in 67%, fatigue in 38%, difficulty in breathing in 19% and muscle pain in 15%.

-How is the evolution of the disease usually?

Most patients have a good prognosis and symptoms disappear within a few days.

In others, however, recovery can take several weeks and become critical and even life threatening.

29. Suspicious cases

-What is considered a suspicious case of COVID-19?

While all people are likely to be infected, there are three cases that are considered highly suspicious:

A patient with acute respiratory infection who has a sudden onset of fever, cough, or shortness of breath, without any other explanatory cause, and with a history of travel or residence in a region reporting local or community transmission of the disease in recent years 14 days.

A patient with any acute respiratory illness who has been in close contact with a confirmed or probable case of COVID-19 in the last 14 days before the onset of symptoms.

A patient with acute respiratory infection with fever, cough, or shortness of breath requiring hospitalization without any other cause to explain this clinical picture.

-What is considered a probable case of COVID-19?

Any suspected case of COVID-19 in which laboratory tests were inconclusive is termed probable.

30. Confirmed cases

-What is considered a confirmed case of COVID-19?

In this way, anyone with positive laboratory confirmation of the virus is considered, regardless of the clinical signs or symptoms that they present.

-And the cases discarded?

They are suspicious cases in which laboratory tests to detect the virus were negative.

31. Most common symptoms of the disease

-What are the most common symptoms of COVID-19?

As we have been discussing the most common signs are fever, cough, sore throat or headache, shortness of breath or difficulty breathing, chills and general discomfort.

There may also be a runny nose and phlegm, although they are rare in these cases.

-What is the severity of these symptoms?

The severity can range from mild to severe. Others, on the other hand, may have the virus and show no signs.

Of the total infected, around 80% recover from the disease without the need for any special treatment.

Of the rest of the cases, about 15% are severe and 5% or critical.

32. Clinical signs to look for

-What clinical signs can indicate the presence of this virus?

In these patients, the amount of circulating platelets in the bloodstream (thrombocytopenia) is frequent, which is considered a bad sign.

For its part, the number of leukocytes in the blood does not provide accurate information about this disease. Both cases of leukopenia (lower than normal) and leukocytosis (increase in number) have been reported.

As for the lymphocyte count, its decrease is more common and usually appears in 80% of patients.

-What inflammatory markers are common in these patients?

The level of procalcitonin in the blood is usually normal at the beginning of the disease but increases in patients who require intensive care.

In severe cases the D-dimer is also elevated.

On the other hand, C-reactive protein (CRP) and the rate of globular sedimentation also increase in the majority of those infected, while in some cases they have elevated liver enzymes, muscle enzymes and myoglobin.

33. Important laboratory tests

-How is COVID-19 diagnosed?

Laboratory tests of samples of the upper respiratory tract (saliva and nasal fluid) and lower (substances from the throat and bronchi) are needed to confirm this disease.

A blood coagulation analysis, another biochemical and a blood count are also usually carried out, together with antibody tests and virus isolation that allow it to be identified and other ailments ruled out.

-What does the PCR test consist of?

This test is known as polymerase chain reaction (PCR). It allows to check if in the cells of a person there are fragments of the genetic material of a certain pathogen or a microorganism causing any illness.

In the particular case of COVID-19, the aim is to detect the presence of a molecule of ribonucleic acid (RNA, the genetic material of the virus). If it appears, it means that the patient is infected.

-What are the advantages and disadvantages of this method?

The PCR test has the advantage that it is very specific, since it allows to differentiate between two very similar pathogens. It is also very effective, because it can detect the virus in the early stages of infection.

On the contrary, its disadvantage is that the results take a couple of hours to come out, which can be a problem in emergencies.

-How is this test performed?

To do this study, you first need to obtain a sample of cells from the patient. To do this, a swab is inserted into both nostrils or to the bottom of the throat and is repeatedly rubbed on the mucosa.

This process is painless although it can cause slight discomfort.

-What are the coronavirus rapid tests?

They are tests that use blood samples to detect the antibodies produced against the disease, or respiratory samples to look for virus proteins.

Unlike PCR, these tests are useful from the fifth day of infection. They also have the disadvantage that they are not as effective and specific.

-How is the quick test performed?

In this case the sample is placed on a test strip with a liquid, which causes the antibodies to be detected.

On the strips some bands appear with the result, as in the pregnancy tests.

-How long does it take to obtain the results of these tests?

In general, the PCR test takes between 4 hours and 6 hours, but due to the high demand as a result of the pandemic, the wait can be as long as two days.

For its part, rapid tests allow results to be obtained in 15 minutes.

-Are the tests one hundred percent effective?

No. The tests can fail, although they are expected to have a reliability greater than 80%.

-What is recommended to do with the results?

If positive, a second test directed at a different SARS-CoV-2 gene is advised to confirm.

In case of negative but persistent suspicion of the disease, it is recommended to take new samples from other sites of the respiratory tract.

-Who should undergo these studies?

People who were listed as suspected cases should undergo these examinations to investigate the presence of SARS-CoV-2 and other respiratory pathogens.

However, due to the growth of the pandemic, it is increasingly recommended that more people undergo these tests. For example, health personnel and other essential services, and especially vulnerable people, such as the elderly in nursing homes, even if they are not serious.

-What controls are usually carried out on people arriving from regions that report local or community transmission of the disease?

People who arrive from affected areas usually have temperature control done at airports with thermal cameras and digital thermometers to detect possible cases of coronavirus.

It is also common for them to respond to a questionnaire and, in cases of suspicion, undergo an evaluation or take them to a hospital for tests.

34. X-rays and chest tomography

-How are the results of chest radiographs in patients with COVID-19?

In the early stages these studies show multiple small irregular shadows and interstitial changes, especially in the peripheral third of the chest, which then progress to bilateral ground glass opacities and pulmonary infiltrates.

In severe cases, lung consolidations and even "blanching" of the lungs are seen. Pleural effusions are rare.

-How are the results of chest CT scans in patients with COVID-19?

In these patients, the virus manifests with bilateral ground glass images and consolidated lung opacities.

Nodular opacities, crazy paving pattern, and a peripheral distribution of the condition may be additional useful features in early diagnosis.

On the other hand, pulmonary cavitation, discrete pulmonary nodules, pleural effusions, and lymphadenopathy are characteristically absent in these patients.

In turn, the follow-up images show a slight or moderate progression of the disease, which is manifested by the increase in the extension and density of the airspace opacities.

-Do these studies serve to diagnose COVID-19?

The use of chest x-rays or computed tomography is not recommended to diagnose this disease, since its results are not specific to this virus. For example, a patient with the flu may have results similar to that of COVID-19.

In turn, the absence of abnormal findings on the initial computed tomography does not rule out the presence of infection by this virus. This may be because incubation takes several days for the infection to cause abnormal examinations.

In any case, although the information provided by these studies is not conclusive, they provide interesting indicators to take into account to accelerate the diagnosis, initiate treatment and isolate patients in cases where necessary.

35. Mild complications

-What are the minor complications suffered by those infected by this virus?

In addition to fever, cough, shortness of breath, and tiredness, infected people may experience headache, sore throat, nasal congestion, and gastrointestinal symptoms such as diarrhea, nausea, and vomiting.

Many patients with COVID-19 suffer from digestive conditions even before respiratory signs.

36. Serious complications

-What are the serious complications suffered by those infected by this virus?

In severe cases many patients suffer from pneumonia (inflammation in the lungs), acute respiratory distress syndrome, septic shock, irreversible metabolic acidosis, and bleeding disorders.

Bronchitis and kidney or other organ failure are also common in this group.

-Who usually suffer from these serious complications?

In general, patients with this type of complications are people over 60 years of age and those with poor immune function.

Also those with respiratory or cardiovascular diseases, diabetes, liver or kidney dysfunction, high blood pressure and some types of cancer.

-Do recovered patients have pulmonary sequelae?

Although it is still too premature to draw conclusions because the disease is very recent, cases have been detected in which the lung is left with some type of fibrosis.

Like this also depends on what was the state of the organ before the disease.

37. Other complications

-What other complications can COVID-19 cause?

This condition can also cause heart damage, even in patients who do not have previous heart conditions.

COVID-19 can cause acute coronary syndromes, arrhythmias, and the development or exacerbation of heart failure.

-What causes this disease in the cardiovascular system?

The virus generates a large inflammation that causes blood clots to form. However, unlike usual heart attacks, thrombosis caused by COVID-19 occurs in very small, microcirculating arteries, in which the catheter cannot be inserted to perform angioplasty

This notably aggravates the picture, since they cannot be uncovered.

Part V. Community-acquired pneumonia

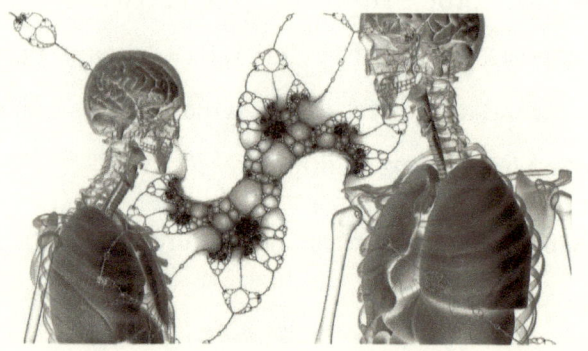

38. Concepts

-Doctor Mario, what is community-acquired pneumonia?

Pneumonia is a respiratory infection in which the air sacs of one or both lungs become inflamed.

The term community acquired is contracted outside of hospitals and other institutions dedicated to health care.

-What are the main symptoms of pneumonia?

The most common signs are chest pain, cough with expectoration, tiredness, high or low fever, chills and tremors, shortness of breath, excessive perspiration, lack of appetite, nausea, vomiting, and diarrhea.

These symptoms can vary from moderate to severe, depending on the type of germ and the general health of the patient.

39. Difference with nosocomial pneumonia

-What is nosocomial pneumonia?

It is the one that is acquired in a hospital or other institutions dedicated to health care.

This type of pneumonia is usually more serious, since the microbes that cause it are more resistant to antibiotics than those found in the community.

Also, because the patients who get it are already sick, they cannot fight them properly.

-Who are more at risk of contracting this type of pneumonia?

Patients who find respirators in intensive care units are at higher risk of contracting this condition.

In addition, it can be transmitted by health workers, who can pass microbes from one patient to another from their bodies, clothes or instruments. So it is of the utmost importance that they wash their hands and use safety and hygiene measures to prevent the spread of germs within the hospital.

Similarly, people who visit loved ones in health centers should also take steps to prevent the spread.

40. Diagnostic criteria

-*What tests are performed to confirm pneumonia?*

If suspected, the doctor will check the lungs with a stethoscope for crackles or abnormal breath sounds. Also, you will surely order a chest x-ray or CT scan.

Other common tests are arterial blood gas, to see if enough oxygen reaches the blood from the lungs; the sputum test, in which samples are taken from the organ in search of microbes; and a blood test, to verify the white blood cell count and confirm the infection.

The doctor may also order a bronchoscopy, in which a flexible tube probe is lowered into the lungs; or a thoracentesis, which draws fluid from the pleural cavity.

-*What are the diagnostic criteria?*

Diagnostic criteria include having started in the community and the presence of the symptoms described above.

Also that the leukocyte count (white blood cells) is greater than 10x10 / L or less than 4 x 10 / L, with or without displacement to the left of the nucleus of neutrophils.

On the other hand, radiographic examination should reveal irregular infiltrates, segmental lobar consolidation, or interstitial changes with or without pleural effusion.

Finally, other non-infectious diseases must be ruled out.

41. Causal pathogenic bacteria

-How is community acquired pneumonia spread?

The most common way is through bacteria, viruses and fungi that are in the air or that are transmitted through droplets emitted by infected people when they cough or sneeze.

Germs are usually prevented by the body from damaging the lungs, but sometimes they are more powerful than the immune system.

-What are the most common pathogenic bacteria and fungi that cause this condition?

Bacteria are the most common cause of pneumonia in adults. The most common is caused by streptococci.

Other bacterial pathogens include *Mycoplasma, Chlamydia, Klebsiella pneumoniae, Escherichia coli, Staphylococcus aureus, Pseudomonas aeruginosa y Acinetobacter baumannii.*

On the other hand, fungal pneumonia is more common in people with chronic health problems or a weakened immune system. These are found in the ground or in the feces of birds, and may vary depending on geographic location.

-What does the treatment of bacterial pneumonia consist of?

Bacterial pneumonia is treated with antibiotics. In addition, the doctor may prescribe cough medicine, fever reducers, and pain relievers.

Generally, people with community-acquired pneumonia can treat their illness from home.

In case of needing hospitalization, the patient will receive intravenous fluids and antibiotics, oxygen therapy and possibly respiratory treatments.

42. Risk factors and prevention

-What are the factors that increase the chances of contracting pneumonia?

We can all suffer from pneumonia, but the disease is more risky in children younger than 2 years and adults older than 65 years.

Factors that increase your chances of getting it include chronic or heart lung disease, liver cirrhosis, diabetes, dementia, stroke, brain injury, and other disorders.

Also smoking cigarettes or having a weakened or suppressed immune system, such as those with HIV / AIDS, those who have had an organ transplant, or those who are receiving chemotherapy.

Also, having undergone recent surgery or trauma increases the risks.

-How can community acquired pneumonia be prevented?

Vaccines can help prevent some types of pneumonia, such as that caused by the flu virus.

On the other hand, it is recommended to avoid smoking, limit alcohol consumption and wash your hands regularly, especially before preparing and consuming food and after going to the bathroom, blowing your nose or changing a baby's diapers.

When coughing or sneezing, it is important to cover your nose and mouth with your arm, tissues, or paper towels to reduce the transmission of drops.

In addition, to maintain a healthy immune system, it is advisable to eat nutritiously, exercise frequently and sleep well.

Lastly, it is important to ventilate interior environments, either with natural ventilation or using exhaust fans.

43. Viral pneumonia

-*What is viral pneumonia?*

It is an inflammation or swelling of the lung tissue caused by a virus. This type of pneumonia is the most common reason for the disease in children under 5 years of age.

-*What are the viruses that cause pneumonia?*

The most common viral pneumonia is caused by the influenza virus.

Other such pathogens include parainfluenza virus, rhinovirus, adenovirus, human metapneumovirus, respiratory syncytial virus, and coronavirus.

-How are viral pneumonias treated?

Unlike bacterial infections, these infections are not treated with antibiotics since they do not destroy viruses. In this case, antivirals are prescribed, especially for the flu.

Treatment may also include corticosteroid medications, increased fluids, oxygen, and use of humidifiers.

44. Pneumonia due to COVID-19

-How is the process by which COVID-19 generates severe pneumonia?

Coronavirus is a respiratory virus, so it begins by infecting the throat. Then once it begins to reproduce, it goes to the bronchial tubes, causing irritation and coughing.

If the situation worsens, it can leave the bronchial canal and reach the lungs, causing inflammation.

When a part of the tissue of this organ is affected, the patient suffers from breathing problems. If the oxygen the body receives is not enough, you should be hospitalized and connected to a respirator.

-What kind of patients affected by COVID-19 suffer from pneumonia?

Most of these patients are older adults or people with chronic lung disease, diabetes, or other chronic conditions.

-What types of symptoms do these patients present?

The most common are fever, cough, and dyspnea. In contrast, in cases that cause pneumonia, signs in the upper respiratory tract are not common.

45. Differences with other pneumonias

-What is the difference between that caused by COVID-19 and other classes of pneumonia?

Unlike bacterial pneumonia, the one caused by COVID-19 cannot be treated with antibiotics and is highly contagious.

Compared to that caused by SARS and MERS, the clinical manifestations and imaging results are similar. However, the one generated by COVID-19 seems to be more infectious.

46. Acute respiratory distress syndrome

-What is acute respiratory distress syndrome?

ARDS is a life-threatening lung condition that prevents sufficient oxygen from reaching the lungs and blood.

-What can cause this ailment?

This syndrome can be caused by any direct or indirect injury to the lung, such as pneumonia, a transplant, septic shock, trauma, or inhalation of vomit or chemicals.

In the case of COVID-19, ARDS develops on average 8 days after the onset of symptoms.

-What causes acute respiratory distress syndrome?

This condition generates an accumulation of fluid in the air sacs (alveoli), which prevents the passage of sufficient oxygen into the bloodstream.

In turn, this fluid also causes the lungs to become heavy and stiff, decreasing their ability to expand.

People with ARDS should receive additional oxygen and generally need the help of a mechanical ventilator to breathe.

-What are the symptoms that this syndrome causes?

The most common signs are shortness of breath, cough, fast heart rate, low blood pressure, rapid breathing, tiredness, fever, and abdominal pain.

-How is acute respiratory distress syndrome treated?

At the moment there is no specific treatment for ARDS. What is sought is to attack the medical problem that caused the injury and provide respiratory support until the lungs heal.

Because most patients need mechanical ventilation, they are generally treated in an intensive care unit.

-What are the results of this treatment?

One in three patients with this disease dies. Of those who survive, most recover their normal lung function, while others suffer permanent damage.

47. Respiratory sepsis and septic shock

-What is respiratory sepsis?

Sepsis is a disease that occurs due to a severe and inflammatory reaction of the body to an infection.

It is not caused by the virus or the invading bacteria, but by the chemicals that the same organism releases into the blood flow to defend against this attack. This generates changes that can damage multiple body systems.

Respiratory sepsis can occur as a consequence of pneumonia.

-What are the symptoms of sepsis?

Faced with a confirmed infection, the signs of this disease are changes in mental status, rapid breathing, chills, dizziness, low blood pressure, and fast heartbeat.

-What is septic shock?

It is a medical condition that occurs when a general infection of the body causes severe low blood pressure.

-In which cases can sepsis progress and cause septic shock?

This occurs when abnormal changes occur in the circulatory system, in the body's cells, and in the way the body uses energy.

Septic shock is a medical emergency and requires urgent attention.

48. Complicaciones extra respiratorias

-What other extra respiratory complications can pneumonia cause?

This disease can cause bacteria that enter the bloodstream from the lungs to spread the infection to other organs and cause organ failure.

On the other hand, pus may form or fluid may accumulate in the cavities of the lungs.

49. Multiple organ failure

-What happens when the infection that causes pneumonia gets worse?

85

Severe cases can lead to respiratory, liver and heart failure.

On the other hand, as sepsis progresses, blood flow to vital organs such as the brain, heart, and kidneys are affected.

In addition, it can lead to the formation of blood clots in the arms, legs, fingers and organs, causing gangrene.

50. Medical discharge for pneumonia

-Is the patient who is discharged for pneumonia fully recovered?

No, the patient usually continues with symptoms despite being discharged. In general, cough, sleep, diet and energy level take between one and two weeks more to return to normal.

-What care should be maintained from home after discharge?

In order to speed recovery and avoid complications, it is recommended to breathe hot and humid air, get plenty of rest, drink plenty of fluids and take medications as prescribed.

In some cases, the use of oxygen may be necessary. Finally, it is important not to smoke or drink alcohol.

Part VI. High risk of mortality

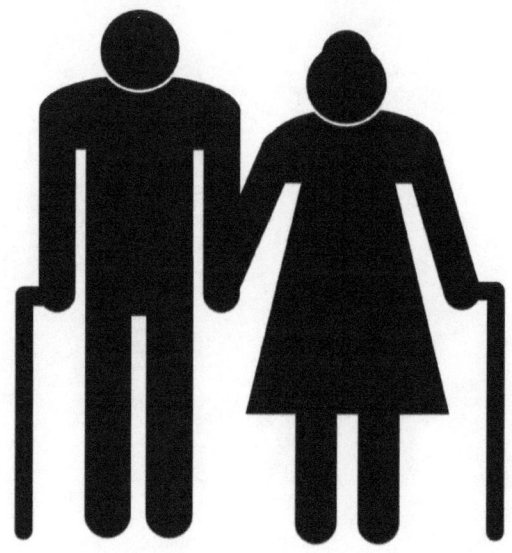

51. Elderly people

-Why are older people more at risk if they become infected with COVID-19?

There are several reasons for this. First, older adults have a weakened immune system that takes longer to respond to infections caused by the virus.

In addition, due to age, they have a greater number of underlying medical conditions that complicate the condition.

On the other hand, the elderly are especially susceptible to respiratory conditions that can cause pneumonia and their lungs are not as resistant as when they were young.

-What are the statistics of mortality from the virus in older adults?

It is estimated that about 15% of patients older than 80 years affected by the virus die. Making a comparison, the number drops to less than one percent in people under 50.

52. Smokers

-What are the health effects of smoking?

Smoking affects most of the body's organs. Among other ailments it can cause cancer, lung diseases, damage and thickening of blood vessels, clots, strokes and vision problems.

Also, smoking during pregnancy increases the risks for both mother and baby.

-Does smoking affect the immune system?

Yes, this vice causes an increase in the concentration of nicotine in the blood, which can generate vasospasm and transient hypoxia in the organs. Furthermore, decreased oxygen in the respiratory tract and viscera damages the immune system and its ability to respond to infections.

-Why does smoking generate more risks in patients with COVID-19?

Along with damage to the immune system, smoking causes continuous and sustained irritation of the airways that favors viral infections, such as COVID-19.

Research in China showed that smokers with the virus are 14 times more likely to progress to pneumonia and suffer from bacterial infections.

On the other hand, the habit of smoking leads to the fingers and cigarettes being in contact with the mouth, which increases the chances of contagion of the virus.

53. Alcoholism

-*What effects does alcoholism have on health?*

Drinking alcohol excessively causes liver disease, such as fatty liver and cirrhosis, and increases the risk of certain types of cancer. It also causes damage to the brain and other organs, and weakens the immune system.

Alcoholism also increases the risks of car accidents, injuries, homicides, and suicides, and is harmful to pregnancy.

-*On social networks, the rumor went viral that drinking alcohol helps prevent the spread of COVID. 19. That's true?*

No, it is totally false. Drinking alcohol does not help or prevent the spread of COVID-19. On the contrary, its consumption is negative, since it decreases the body's defense capacity and damages the organs.

54. Bronchial asthma

-What is asthma?

Asthma is a disease that causes the airways to swell and narrow, producing more mucus. This can lead to shortness of breath, shortness of breath, cough, and wheezing.

-What causes asthma?

Asthma occurs when swelling of the airways occurs. This can be caused by inhaling certain substances found in the air, such as pollen, dust mites, mold, dandruff, or fur from pets.

In addition, it can also be triggered by stressful situations, exercise, cold air or the consumption of certain medications.

-Why are asthmatics more at risk compared to COVID-19?

Asthma makes the airways more susceptible to infections, especially those caused by viruses. These tend to generate greater bronchial inflammation in these patients, inducing bronchial hyperresponsiveness and an increased risk of asthmatic crisis.

-What should asthmatics do in front of COVID-19?

It is important that these patients follow the treatment prescribed by their doctors to control asthma. This includes applying your preventive inhaler dose every day to reduce your risk of having a seizure.

Otherwise, mild bronchial inflammation may make them more susceptible to respiratory infections.

They should also follow preventive care common to everyone, such as frequent hand washing.

-How do the symptoms of an asthma crisis differ from those caused by COVID-19?

Infection caused by COVID-19 usually includes fever, cough, and shortness of breath, while asthma usually does not include fever and is characterized by wheezing, a high-pitched sound as air passes through the airways.

55. Cardiovascular diseases

-What is cardiovascular disease?

It is a term used to describe problems with the heart and blood vessels. This includes ailments such as coronary heart disease, heart failure, arrhythmias, heart valve conditions, stroke, hypertension, and congenital heart disease, among others.

-Why are patients with this type of disease at greater risk compared to COVID-19?

This is due to the multiple direct and indirect complications that the virus can cause, such as acute myocardial damage, myocarditis, arrhythmias, and venous thromboembolism.

In turn, many of the treatments being used to control COVID-19 also have negative cardiac side effects.

On the other hand, it has been discovered that the virus can cause damage to the heart, even in patients who had no previous conditions. This is because it generates a large inflammation that causes blood clots to form.

56. Chronic lung disease

-What is chronic lung disease?

It is any common condition in the lungs that affects the capacity of lungs to work properly. It includes diseases in the airways that transport oxygen, in the lung tissue and in the blood vessels of this organ.

-*Why are people with chronic lung disease more at risk compared to COVID-19?*

These patients are more likely to have inflammation in the lungs and high blood pressure in the arteries that carry blood to these organs.

In addition, these ailments increase the risks of attack and heart failure and of suffering from lung cancer.

57. Diabetes mellitus

-*What is diabetes mellitus?*

Diabetes mellitus or type 2 diabetes is a chronic disorder that prevents the proper metabolism of glucose, causing it to accumulate in the blood.

This can be caused by a deficit in the production of insulin in the pancreas or by a resistance of the cells to this hormone.

This condition affects both adults and children and, if left untreated, can lead to long-term damage to the heart, blood vessels, and kidneys, eye problems, polyneuropathies, and severe foot ulcers.

-Why are people with diabetes more at risk compared to COVID-19?

This is because coronavirus infection may be more difficult to treat as a result of fluctuations in blood glucose levels.

In addition, the immune system is affected, making it difficult to fight the virus.

On the other hand, diabetes can generate other complications, such as heart disease and stroke, kidney damage, and nerve damage that further complicate the condition.

58. Chronic kidney disease

-What is chronic kidney disease?

It is a disease that involves the gradual loss of kidney function.

These organs are responsible for filtering waste and excess fluids in the form of urine. They are also responsible for balancing the salts and minerals that circulate in the blood, such as calcium, phosphorus, sodium, and potassium, and help control blood pressure.

-Why are people with chronic kidney disease more at risk compared to COVID-19?

These patients present more risks because the disease involves a state of immune deficiency and associated ailments, such as anemia, changes in sugar levels, cardiovascular problems, liver damage, and pulmonary edema.

In turn, people who need hemodialysis spend more time in transport and closed sanitary spaces, which favors contagion and health complications.

59. Hypothyroidism

-What is hypothyroidism?

Hypothyroidism is a disease in which the thyroid does not make enough thyroid hormone. This gland is one of the most important in the body and its activity influences metabolism and most of the bodily functions, such as heart rate and blood pressure.

That there are usual levels of this hormone in the body is essential for normal growth and development in childhood, and for the functioning of the brain throughout life.

-Why are people with hypothyroidism more at risk compared to COVID-19?

These patients are believed to be more at risk since their main cause is Hashimoto's Disease, an autoimmune condition in which the immune system itself attacks healthy cells in the body by mistake.

Moreover, at the moment there are no concrete data to confirm that patients with this type of disease are at greater risk of developing more serious complications of COVID-19.

However, if it is not treated properly, hypothyroidism can cause infections, heart problems and peripheral neuropathy, among other complications that can hinder the patient's general picture, so it is important to increase care.

60. Adrenal insufficiency

-What is adrenal insufficiency?

It is a condition that occurs when the adrenal glands do not make enough hormones.

It is a rare disorder that can affect anyone of any age and, if left untreated, can lead to death. It is usually caused by a problem with the immune system.

Among other essential functions, the hormones produced by the adrenal glands allow normal growth and regulate metabolism, energy levels, blood pressure, and stress response.

-Why are people with adrenal insufficiency more at risk compared to COVID-19?

These patients often take glucocorticoids, drugs that mimic the effects of hormones the body naturally produces in the adrenal glands.

This can make them more susceptible to COVID-19 because these drugs suppress the immune system. Furthermore, they may also experience more serious illness, as glucocorticoids suppress their own steroid response to infection.

On the other hand, these patients are at risk of suffering an adrenal crisis, as a consequence of very low levels of cortisol in the blood. This causes diarrhea, vomiting, dehydration and a drop in sugar in the body that require immediate attention.

Furthermore, people with this condition generally suffer from associated autoimmune diseases, such as diabetes, chronic thyroiditis, hypoparathyroidism, testicular failure, pernicious anemia, and hyperthyroidism, which makes COVID-19 more severe.

61. Obesity

-*What is obesity?*

Obesity is a chronic disease characterized by the excessive accumulation of fat in the body, which produces a clear increase in risk to the person's health.

Someone is considered obese when the percentage of fat exceeds 25% of body weight in men and 33% in women.

-Why are people with obesity more at risk compared to COVID-19?

These patients are more at risk since obesity causes a chronic inflammatory state and an increase in cardiovascular and respiratory diseases, in addition to diabetes, hypertension and sleep apnea, which increase the severity of COVID-19.

62. HIV / AIDS

-What is HIV?

Human immunodeficiency virus (HIV) is a virus that is transmitted sexually, through the blood or through breast milk, and causes AIDS, a disease that weakens the immune system.

When a person contracts this virus, it remains within the body for life.

This condition is treated with drugs that prevent the virus from reproducing.

-Why are people with HIV / AIDS more at risk compared to COVID-19?

Because this virus damages the immune system, these patients have a higher risk of contracting infections. However, studies to date do not indicate that people with HIV and a strong immune system are more likely to be affected by COVID-19 or that the infection progresses more severely.

In any case, it is necessary to expand research on this topic.

63. Malignant tumors

-What are malignant tumors?

Malignant or carcinogenic tumor is a disease characterized by the transformation of cells, which proliferate rapidly and uncontrollably and do not die normally due to changes in their genetic structure.

-Why are people with malignant tumors more at risk compared to COVID-19?

These patients are more at risk because treatments for this disease, especially chemotherapy, often weaken the immune system, reducing the ability to fight infection.

-Do patients who receive hormonal therapies for breast or ovarian cancer have a higher risk of contracting COVID-19 or having a more serious disease?

Currently, there is no evidence that hormonal therapies can increase the risk of contracting COVID-19 or having a more serious disease. Most of these therapies do not suppress the immune system.

64. Transplanted

-Why are transplant recipients more at risk compared to COVID-19?

This is because they take immunosuppressants, a medication that reduces the risk of rejection of the transplanted organ, but that lowers the defenses.

In turn, these patients are in a moment of special vulnerability after a transplant.

65. Use of steroids

-What are steroids?

Anabolic steroids are male sex hormones, or synthetic substances based on them, that are used for different purposes.

Within the field of medicine, they are used to treat hormonal problems, late puberty and the loss of muscle mass as a consequence of different diseases.

In sports and athletics, they are used to improve performance. However, its consumption is illegal and can generate serious health problems.

-What unwanted effects can its use generate?

Steroids can cause serious heart problems, including heart attack, and the development of liver or testicular tumors.

Other unwanted effects are infertility, severe acne, increased blood pressure, aggressive and violent behavior, abnormal cholesterol levels, psychiatric disorders, and drug dependence.

-Why are people taking steroids more at risk compared to COVID-19?

These substances have been shown to affect the immune system's ability to fight COVID-19 and other infections.

Also, people who consume them take longer to remove the virus from their bodies.

66. Immunosuppressed

-*What is an immunosuppressed patient?*

He is a patient whose immune system works below the normal index, making him more susceptible to infections.

This condition can be a consequence of HIV / AIDS, leukemia, diabetes, an organ transplant, cancer, malnutrition, the use of certain medications and certain genetic disorders, among other possibilities.

-*Why are immunodepressed people more at risk compared to COVID-19?*

These patients have a higher risk of contracting viral infections such as COVID-19, since their ability to fight them is diminished.

67. Mentally ill and disabled

-Why are the mentally ill and the disabled more at risk compared to COVID-19?

These people are at risk because, although they may not have a specific health problem, they have greater care needs.

Mandatory isolation measures and the saturation of health systems stemming from the COVID-19 pandemic endanger these vulnerable publics, who in many cases depend on social and personal assistance.

Social distancing can leave unprotected those who, for example, require support to eat, dress or take a bath.

Part VII. Global and community epidemiology

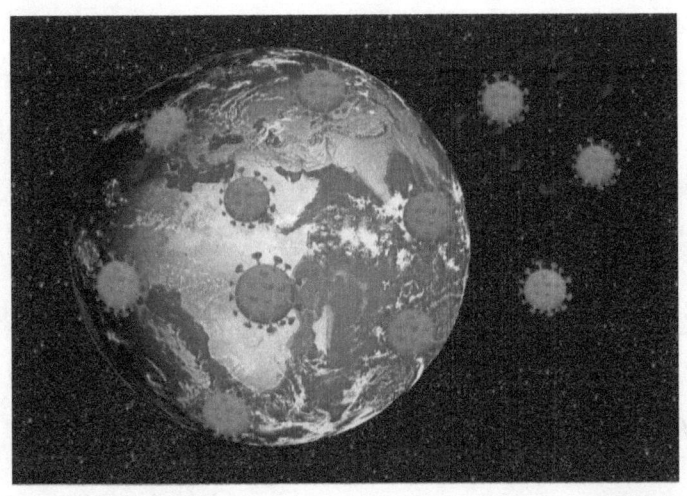

68. Epidemics in the history of humanity

-What other epidemics did humanity face before COVID-19?

Epidemics have been a constant throughout history, even since the Ancient Age.

Among the most lethal are the Justinian Plague (541-542), the Black Death (1346-1353), Smallpox (1520), the Spanish Flu (1918-1920) and HIV / AIDS (1981-present), each of which caused between 25 and 50 million deaths.

We can also name the Antonine Plague (165-180), the Third Plague (1855), the Russian Flu (1889-1890) Cholera (1817-1923), the Asian Flu (1957-1958) and the Hong Kong Flu (1968-1970).

Finally, among the most recent are swine flu (2009-2010), Ebola (2014-2016) and those caused by coronaviruses.

69. Previous coronavirus epidemics

-What were the previous epidemics caused by coronaviruses?

Before the current one, two cases were registered. The first to appear was severe acute respiratory syndrome (SARS-CoV), between November 2002 and July 2003. It started in southern China and ended with infected people in 17 countries, although most cases were recorded in China and Hong Kong; it caused 800 deaths, with a lethality of 9.6%.

The second was the Middle East respiratory syndrome (MERS-CoV), in June 2012. The first case was registered in Saudi Arabia and then spread to 27 countries in Asia, Europe, Africa and North America. It was more lethal than the previous one (34.5%) and caused 850 deaths.

70. Start, development and end of the pandemic

-What are the phases of a pandemic?

The pandemic is an epidemic outbreak that affects everyone. According to the World Health Organization, it is divided into 7 phases.

In the first, the virus circulates between animals and transmission to humans is not reported.

In the second, the virus present in domestic and wild animals infects humans.

In the third phase, small groups of people acquire the infection. Contagion occurs in a limited way and under specific circumstances. The fact that the virus is transmitted between humans does not necessarily mean that it will cause a pandemic.

In the fourth, transmission between people is verified and the virus generates outbreaks of the disease in communities. At this stage, there is an increased risk of a pandemic breaking out, but it does not necessarily mean that it is coming.

In the fifth, the virus is spread among humans in at least two countries in the same region. At this stage the pandemic is imminent and the time for measures to mitigate the infection are short.

In the sixth pandemic occurs and the disease spreads in different regions of the world.

In the seventh the virus reaches its peak and the disease levels are reduced. However, it is uncertain whether further waves will occur in the future.

71. Possibilities of local endemics

-What is a local endemic?

The endemic refers to the condition of an infectious disease that permanently or on a regular date affects a specific country or region.

It results in a condition that persists for a time in a specific place, attacking a significant number of people. However, the figure does not vary dramatically and is always stable.

The disease may or may not be serious and at some point it may become an epidemic.

-What is the cause of these endemics?

Generally they occur due to economic, cultural, social, ecological and biological factors.

For example, they may be due to the lack of prevention, basic sanitation and water control, to certain climatic conditions that favor contagion or the susceptibility of people, among other possibilities.

-What are some examples of endemic diseases?

Among them we can mention malaria, Chagas disease, dengue, yellow fever, tuberculosis and whooping cough, which attack certain regions of the world.

72. Local, national and international measures

-What measures are recommended at the local level to stop the pandemic?

The recommendation at the local level is that people stay home, stay away from the sick and limit face-to-face contact with others as much as possible.

This also includes avoiding shaking hands, hugging or kissing others, and not visiting vulnerable audiences, such as those in nursing homes or hospitals, babies, or people with compromised immune systems.

In addition, citizens are advised to consult health care centers in cases of COVID-19 risk and to follow general care to prevent infection, such as frequent hand washing.

Regarding the use of face masks, the instructions recommended by the local public health provider should be followed.

-What measures are recommended at the national level to stop the pandemic?

When the virus occurs nationwide, authorities can implement social distancing measures to reduce the potential for transmission of the disease.

This may include general quarantines with the closing of factories, offices, banks, schools, theaters, cinemas, shopping malls, restaurants, gyms and non-essential shops, and the suspension of sporting, cultural and social events and events.

Also the closing of borders and the prohibition to go out without a justification.

The implementation of these practices requires broad community participation and continuous and transparent public health communications.

-What measures are recommended at the international level to stop the pandemic?

From the international level, humanitarian aid and joint work are expected to control the disease and find a cure.

However, except for the general recommendations of the World Health Organization, at the moment only individual responses from the countries have been seen based on their own interests and needs, and it has not been possible to address the issue globally, with measures community.

The pandemic poses a global crisis scenario that, in addition to health, is also economic as a result of the paralysis of activities.

For this reason, the measures taken at the international level must include aid and collaboration in both areas.

73. Quarantine and social isolation

-What is a quarantine?

Quarantine is preventive isolation that a person or animal is subjected to for a period of time, for health reasons.

It applies to those who were exposed to a contagious disease, but who did not necessarily become infected. The objective is to check during this process if the person shows signs of the illness or not.

-What is quarantine and social isolation for?

These measures serve to decrease the chain of contagion. By lowering the number of infected people, vulnerable publics are protected and the need for hospital care is reduced, preventing the collapse of the health system.

-Why are COVID-19 quarantine periods of 14 days?

This is because the maximum time that elapses between a person's infection and the onset of disease symptoms is 14 days.

This prevents infected people without signs from continuing to transmit the disease to others without knowing it.

74. Individual protection for the sick

-What should a person do if he/she thinks he/she is infected with COVID-19?

In that case the person should immediately contact the local institution designated for the evaluation, diagnosis and treatment of the disease.

Unless you need urgent medical attention, you will most likely be recommended to isolate yourself at home and manage your symptoms.

-What protection measures should be taken in these cases?

As much as possible, this patient should be kept away from other people and pets in the house. Also, you should not receive visits or leave your home unless you need urgent care.

In case of living with others, when they are in the same room you will have to use a chinstrap that covers your mouth, as long as this does not hinder your breathing.

Ideally, if conditions permit, you should stay in a separate room from the rest and use a different bathroom. It is also recommended that you use your own dishes, glasses, cutlery, bedding and towels, and that you do not share them with others.

When coughing or sneezing, you should do so in a disposable tissue and immediately wash your hands with soap and water.

-In which cases should you call a doctor?

If the condition worsens and the patient has trouble breathing, a high fever, or is confused or drowsy, seek medical attention.

75. Individual protection of your contacts

-What should the close contacts of a patient do with COVID-19?

These people also have to isolate themselves, quarantine and avoid contact with others.

In case of living in the same house as the infected, if the patient cannot use a chinstrap, the caregivers must do so while they are in the same room.

Additionally, they are encouraged to ventilate shared spaces, either by opening a window or turning on an air filter.

On the other hand, like the rest of the people, they must follow the protection measures, such as washing their hands frequently and disinfecting the objects that are touched the most, such as mobile phones, light switches, remote controls and door handles.

When touching and washing the patient's clothes, sheets and towels, it is advisable to wear gloves and use hot water and detergent.

-How long should these contacts be kept isolated?

These people should be kept isolated for 14 days from the last contact with the confirmed case.

In case of living in the same home, 14 days must pass from the last day in which this patient presented symptoms.

76. Protection of health personnel

-*What protection measures should health personnel follow?*

These workers must follow strict hygiene and infection control regulations to reduce the risks of transmission.

This includes personal protection measures, disinfection of environments and correct waste management.

-*What kind of protection should they use when dealing with infected patients?*

Protection includes the use of special clothing, such as caps, surgical medical masks, latex gloves, a waterproof long-sleeved gown, disposable shoe covers, and anti-splash lenses.

In addition, they must follow strict hand hygiene before and after contact with the patient and upon entering and leaving the hospital.

-How is the treatment of hospital waste?

The waste follows a decontamination, collection and disposal protocol that is similar to that used for other types of similar microorganisms.

These wastes are considered Class III or as Special Biosanitary wastes.

77. Protection of security personnel

-What protection measures must the security personnel follow?

In case of being in contact with infected patients, they must follow similar protection measures as those of health personnel.

In the event of not maintaining specific contact, they must follow the general prevention and care recommendations valid for the entire population.

78. Declaration of cessation of quarantine

- *When is the cessation of quarantine declared?*

As we have been explaining, the quarantine for close contacts and suspected cases lasts 14 days.

In the cases of the general quarantines that many countries are imposing on all their citizens, they end when the time of preventive isolation established by the health authorities passes.

Once finished, the return to activities is carried out gradually, taking special care of the most vulnerable audiences.

-*When does a COVID-19 patient receive a medical discharge?*

To be discharged, these patients must be stable and fever free, and the lung images must show significant improvement with no signs of organ dysfunction.

Furthermore, breathing and speech must be normalized and the person must be in clear consciousness for at least 3 days.

Finally, they must have two consecutive negative results carried out on different days of the PCR test, which detects the presence of ribonucleic acid, the genetic material of the virus.

79. Declaration of cessation of transmission

-What are the criteria to declare the end of the transmission of a virus?

The criteria depend on each case in particular, by virtue of the characteristics of the virus, the form of infection, the people infected, their development and treatment, among other factors.

For example, in the case of Ebola virus, the outbreak was terminated after 42 days had elapsed since the last confirmed case was negative twice in a row in blood tests carried out to detect its presence.

These 42 days were equivalent to twice the maximum incubation period of the infection. Therefore, after that period it was possible to confirm the interruption of the transmission of the disease from person to person.

Regarding the new coronavirus, the criteria applied are not yet known.

80. Notifiable disease

-What are notifiable diseases?

These are diseases that are considered of great importance for public health and the country's health authorities require doctors, laboratories and hospital institutions to notify them when they are diagnosed. COVID-19 is among these diseases.

-What is the purpose of this notification?

Their communication allows to know statistical data on the disease. This is very helpful for researchers to track their outbreaks, understand how they spread, and control it.

Part VIII. Prevention of disease

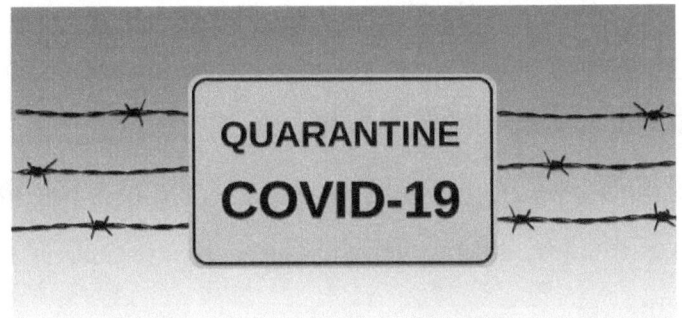

81. Surveillance for symptom-free contacts

-Doctor Mario, do asymptomatic or mild signs need to be hospitalized?

No. Patients who do not have symptoms or in whom they are very mild - a little cough, fever below 38 degrees, nasal congestion, general discomfort - do not need to be hospitalized and can recover and quarantine at home.

Hospitalization should only be evaluated if they are people with chronic health problems or have a weakened immune system.

-What is the surveillance that these patients must follow at home?

These patients should control fever and contact a doctor in cases where it is above 38 degrees, or when they have difficulty breathing, constant chest pain or pressure, changes in mental state, confusion, trouble waking up or a bluish tint to the lips or face.

82. Caring for the patient with COVID-19 at home

-*What care should be taken with a coronavirus patient at home?*

Whenever possible, the patient should be kept in a separate room and not receive visits or leave the home unless his symptoms worsen.

When in the presence of other people, you should cover yourself with a chinstrap and keep a distance of more than two meters. When coughing or sneezing, you should do so in a disposable tissue and immediately wash your hands with soap and water.

On the other hand, it is important to ventilate shared spaces, either by opening a window or turning on an air filter, and limiting the number of caregivers. For this task, the ideal is to appoint a young person who is in good health and does not have chronic diseases.

In addition, the patient must use different dishes, glasses, cutlery, bedding and towels.

Finally, objects that are frequently touched must be disinfected and all the inhabitants of the house must follow the general care for the disease, such as washing their hands and avoiding touching their eyes, nose and mouth.

83. Transfer of suspects or sick

-What should be done if a suspicious or sick patient needs to be transferred?

Transportation should be in specially designated vehicles, where possible negative pressure ambulances. These cars must be disinfected frequently.

On the other hand, both the patient's companion and medical personnel should wear a mask and protective suits to avoid contagion.

-What are negative pressure ambulances?

They are ambulances with technical means that allow the air pressure inside the vehicle to be lower than the outside pressure. In this way, the air can be filtered and purified before its emission, minimizing the possibilities of virus infection and transmission.

84. Complicated hospitalization

-In which patients with COVID-19 is hospitalization recommended?

Hospitalization is recommended for those with a severe or serious illness, or with associated chronic health problems.

By severe disease is meant patients who have a respiratory rate of more than 30 breaths per minute; a blood oxygen saturation of less than 93 percent; a Kirby or PaO2 / FiO2 index (which indirectly measures lung injury) less than 300; and pulmonary infiltrates (characteristic of an infection) greater than 50 percent in 24-48 hours.

Meanwhile, the seriously ill are those with respiratory failure who need mechanical ventilation or septic shock.

85. Conjunctural hospitalization centers

-How is the management of patients with COVID-19 in hospitalization centers?

Ideally, these patients should be isolated in individual rooms. If this is not possible due to the limited number of rooms, it is acceptable to group people with COVID-19 in the same place, always keeping a minimum distance of 1.5 meters between the beds.

In suspicious cases, the results of the tests must be awaited before placing them in these shared rooms, since many may have other respiratory diseases not related to this virus.

-What conditions should these isolation rooms have?

These spaces must have adequate materials for hand washing and hygiene, ventilation, appropriate waste containers and indicator signs on the door and inside, indicating that it is an isolation zone.

On the other hand, specific hygiene and disinfection measures must be taken and entry should be allowed only to authorized personnel.

-How do you avoid contagion in hospital centers?

In these centers, strict hygiene and infection control regulations must be followed to reduce the risks of transmission. This includes personal protection measures, hand hygiene, environmental disinfection and waste management, among other actions.

On the other hand, anyone visiting these hospitals should wear a mask and avoid close contact with patients with symptoms of respiratory diseases. They should also wash their hands with soap or alcohol-based disinfectant, cover their nose and mouth with disposable tissues when coughing or sneezing, and follow the rest of the preventive care in these cases.

86. Intensive care and assisted ventilation

-How is the treatment against COVID-19?

There are currently no specific vaccines or antiviral treatments against this virus. However, patients may receive medical attention to alleviate symptoms. Most of those infected with the virus recover with the help of these support measures.

-What is the care provided to these patients?

When the patient is admitted, he is placed on a bed in rest and kept well hydrated and balanced, constantly monitoring his vital signs and oxygen saturation.

Blood, urine, C-reactive protein (PCR), biochemical indicators, and coagulation function tests are usually performed to check that they are within normal parameters.

Arterial blood gas analysis and imaging tests of the chest are also performed periodically.

-What is the treatment in case of changes in oxygen saturation?

When this value is less than 90 percent, supplemental oxygen therapy is applied, which may include a nasal catheter, an oxygen mask, high-flow transnasal oxygen therapy, and non-invasive or invasive mechanical ventilation, among other possibilities.

In cases where hypoxemic acute respiratory failure does not respond to conventional treatment, a high-flow nasal cannula (HFNC) and non-invasive positive pressure ventilation (NIPPV) can be used.

87. General and immunological support measures

-What are the general and immunological support measures that are followed with these patients?

As I mentioned, these patients are regularly monitored to identify and treat complications associated with the virus, such as acute respiratory distress syndrome (ARDS), sepsis or septic shock.

There are cases in which they are offered oxygen therapy, fluid replacement or antibacterial treatments. Antivirals and other associated therapies are also tested in some patients.

-What are you looking for with these measures?

This seeks to attack the two main components of the disease. On the one hand, the viral infection itself, for which certain drugs are being tested, and on the other, when pneumonia progresses, severe inflammation of the lungs, which is tried to control with drugs for the immune and inflammatory process.

88. Antivirals, Antibiotics, and Steroids

-Is there any medicine to prevent or treat COVID-19 infection?

At the moment, no specific medication is recommended to prevent or treat this disease. However, some treatments are being studied and there are several clinical trials underway to test their efficacy.

-Are antibiotics effective in treating COVID-19?

No. Antibiotics are only effective against bacterial infections. This disease is caused by a virus, so these drugs do not work against it.

However, during hospitalization the patient may receive antibiotics to prevent them from contracting secondary bacterial infections.

-Is there any effective antiviral therapy against COVID-19?

At the moment there is no proven antiviral therapy that works against this virus. However, multiple tests are underway to analyze the use of various medications.

Preliminary studies with some of these drugs have shown a reduction in the viral load in patients affected by COVID-19. However, the evidence is not yet definitive and more research is needed.

-What are the medications being tested?

Among them are chloroquine and hydroxychloroquine, two antimalarials that are also used to treat autoimmune diseases such as lupus and some types of arthritis.

Also remdesivir, an experimental drug originally developed to treat the Ebola virus; and lopinavir / ritonavir, a combination of antiretrovirals that are used for HIV.

Other tests are with interferon Beta b1, a molecule produced by the body itself to fight viral infections and which helps regulate inflammation; and with colchicine, a powerful anti-inflammatory agent used in the treatment and prevention of gout and Familial Mediterranean Fever.

Other drugs being studied are oseltamivir, ribavirin, penciclovir, nitazoxanide, nafamostat, tocilizumab, azithromycin, corticosteroids, and IV immunoglobulin.

-Why are old antiviral drugs used as evidence in these treatments?

This measure is especially effective since these are remedies for which the safety profile, side effects, dosage and pharmacological interactions are known, which would facilitate their implementation if they are effective.

-What are corticosteroids?

Corticosteroids are medications similar to hormones that are produced by the adrenal glands. They serve to reduce inflammation and in many cases affect the immune system.

They are generally very powerful drugs that cause side effects, for which in case of use they are usually indicated for short periods of time.

-In which cases of COVID-19 is the use of corticosteroids suggested?

These medications are recommended for patients with acute respiratory distress syndrome receiving mechanical ventilation. However, its effectiveness as part of therapy against COVID-19 has not yet been definitively confirmed.

89. Current and future vaccines

-Is there currently a vaccine against COVID-19?

No. At the moment there is no vaccine against this virus.

-Do pneumonia vaccines protect against this disease?

No. Pneumonia vaccines, such as pneumococcal and Haemophilus influenzae type B (Hib) vaccine, do not protect against the new coronavirus.

However, even though they are not effective against COVID-19, many patients are advised to take them to maintain good health.

-How long could it take to develop a vaccine against COVID-19?

It is estimated that its development can take between 6 months and a year and a half.

The terms are generally much longer, but it is possible that in this global crisis situation there will be more flexibility for international regulatory bodies to approve.

90. Control of chronic patients

-How is the control of chronic patients in times of COVID-19?

These patients must take extreme care since the virus is usually more serious in those who suffer from chronic diseases.

During this period it is recommended that they avoid going to hospitals and that they only do so in emergencies, to reduce the risks of infection.

For example, many regular check-ups for your ailments can be done remotely, consulting the doctor over the phone or via video conference.

In cases where it is necessary to go to a hospital center, it is important that they set a prior schedule to limit the time of the visit and take all available protective measures.

91. Vitamins and nutrition

-What nutritional care is recommended during the COVID-19 outbreak?

During this period, it is especially important to have a balanced diet and eat protein-rich foods such as fish, meat, eggs, milk, legumes and nuts on a daily basis. Also fresh fruits and vegetables. Also, you should drink at least a liter and a half of water per day.

-What foods should be avoided during the pandemic?

During this time it is recommended to avoid fasting, dieting and eating raw food, meat of wild animals or little known products.

-*Are vitamin supplements recommended?*

While the pandemic lasts, the diet can be supplemented with multivitamins, minerals and deep-sea fish oil.

On the other hand, vitamin D supplementation could help prevent acute respiratory infections.

92. Management of social and individual stress

-*What is stress?*

Stress is a feeling of tiredness and physical or emotional tension that arises in response to a difficult situation, demand or thought to cope.

It can cause various mental and physical disorders, as well as frustration, anger and nervousness.

-*What are its effects?*

Its most common effects are headaches and chest pain, muscle tension, fatigue, changes in sexual desire, upset stomach and sleep problems.

In turn, it can also affect mood and generate anxiety, restlessness, lack of motivation, irritability, anger and sadness.

Another consequence is compulsive behaviors, such as excessive food consumption, drug addiction, alcoholism, and smoking.

-What can I do to manage stress during quarantine?

Quarantine inevitably generates a quota of tension, since it implies a change in routine and a new and uncertain situation.

In this framework it is important to maintain daily customs as much as possible, such as the times we get up, eat and go to sleep.

Another key point is not to isolate yourself. Even at a distance it is vital to stay connected with family and friends, whether through calls, messages or video conferences. Links are a great shock absorber for stress and help us not feel lonely.

On the other hand, it is recommended to practice relaxation techniques, eat healthy, do physical activity, rest properly and avoid drug and alcohol abuse.

-What can we do not to panic during the pandemic?

In addition to the aforementioned, we must dose the amount of information to which we are exposed.

During these situations, many alarmist news and false rumors tend to spread, which can generate a greater feeling of fear, anxiety and anguish. Therefore, it is important to stay informed through reliable means and only a few times a day so as not to get saturated.

Finally, it is essential to focus on recreational and enjoyable activities, such as listening to music, reading or watching movies, to keep your head busy and with positive thoughts.

-What are the recommendations to help young children at this stage?

Children's reactions will depend largely on the actions of the parents. If adults are nervous and tense, they will pass it on to their children. Therefore it is important to stay calm and create a feeling of calm.

Children should not be hidden from what is happening. Rather, the situation needs to be explained to them in the right words and tone for their respective ages.

In addition, during this time it is key to maintain family routines as much as possible and encourage them to carry out recreational and recreational activities that help them express their feelings in a positive way.

In this type of situation it is normal for children to look for more attachment and to be more demanding with their parents, so it is necessary to arm yourself with patience and be understanding.

93. Natural and traditional treatments

-*Are there any natural or traditional treatments that prevent or cure COVID-19?*

At the moment there is no evidence of therapies of this type that cure or prevent the disease.

However, some natural or traditional treatments can help alleviate some of the symptoms caused by COVID-19.

-What Chinese herbs in common use have been used against this virus?

Some of the herbal formulas used were rizoma phragmitis (lu gen), rizoma imperatae (baimao gen), radix angelicae dahuricae (baizhi), rizoma atractylodis macrocephalae (baizhu), rizoma atractylodis (cangzhu), madreselva (jinyininel) hua), herba pogostemonis (huoxiang), radix et rizoma rhodiolae crenulatae (hongjingtian), rizoma dryopteridiscrassi rhizomatis (guanzhong), rizoma polygonicuspidati (huzhang), fructustsaoko (cao gutaciu), foliummori (sang ye), radix astragali praeparata (huangqi), radix ligustici brachylobi (fang feng) and herba eupatorii (peilan).

However, these types of formulas should only be used under the guidance of specialized doctors.

- Can eating garlic help prevent COVID-19?

Garlic is a healthy food that can have certain antimicrobial properties. However, at the moment there is no evidence that eating it helps prevent this condition.

Part IX. Individual and collective protection

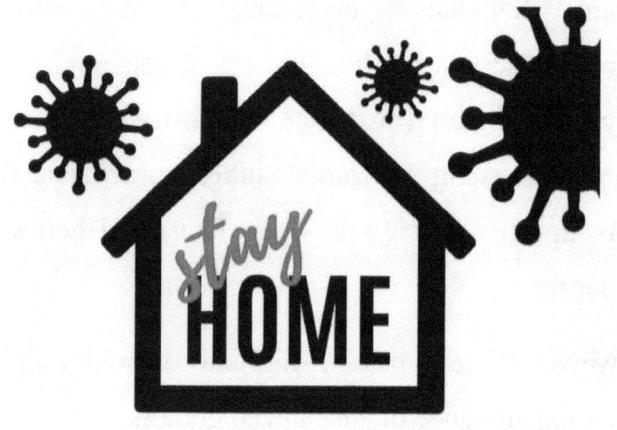

94. Weather care

-*Doctor Mario, is it true that COVID-19 cannot be transmitted in areas with very hot climates?*

No. The research carried out so far indicates that the virus can be transmitted in any region, including those in hot and humid climates. Therefore, it is important to take all the necessary protection and care measures, regardless of the climatic conditions of the place where you live.

-*Is it true that exposure to sunlight or high temperatures prevents contagion?*

No. This is also false. The virus can be contracted even on very hot and hot days.

- *Can exposure to intense cold and snow kill the virus?*

No. In general, the human body maintains its temperature around 36.5 and 37 degrees, regardless of the outside temperature or the weather conditions of the place where the person is. So there is no point in exposing yourself to intense cold or snow.

-*Does bathing with hot water prevent infection with COVID-19?*

No. Bathing in hot water does not provide any protection against the virus. Body temperature will also remain the same regardless of the water temperature.

95. Use and type of masks

-Is it necessary to wear masks permanently to protect yourself from COVID-19?

Initially, the recommendation was the use of masks by those who present symptoms of the disease or are not caring for or in contact with a sick person, without the need for use by the entire community. However, recently due to the high number of infections, several agencies such as the FDA in the United States, recommend the use of masks and even homemade chinstraps for protection.

These masks are disposable and can only be used once, so it is important to use them rationally to prevent them from running out.

-What is the correct way to use these masks?

Before touching the mask, wash your hands with soap and water or with an alcohol-based disinfectant. Then you have to carefully inspect it for tears or holes.

When laying, the correct side should be oriented outwards, which is generally colored. It must cover both the mouth and chin and the nose.

The chinstrap should be changed as soon as it is wet. When discarding it, the elastic tapes must be removed from behind the ears, away from the face and clothing to avoid touching potentially contaminated surfaces. Then it should be thrown into a closed container.

Finally, after handling, you must wash your hands again.

-How many types of masks are there?

There are 3 main types. Some are the N95 / KN95 respirators, which filters 95 % of the particles with an aerodynamic diameter greater than or equal to 0.3 μm.

Others are disposable surgical masks, which have 3 layers of protection. The external one prevents drops from entering the mask, the internal one has a filter to block 90 percent of the particles with a diameter greater than 5 μm, and the internal one in contact with the nose and mouth absorbs moisture.

Finally there are the cotton chinstraps, which are heavy and do not fit well on the face, so they are not very effective against viruses.

-When should a mask be replaced?

All types of masks must be replaced on a regular basis. Especially when it is difficult to breathe through it, when it is damaged, when it cannot adjust correctly to the contour of the face, when it is contaminated with blood or respiratory drops or after maintaining contact with an infected patient.

96. Hand washing

-Why is it important to wash your hands frequently to prevent contagion?

Hand washing is key because when it is done with soap and water or using an alcohol-based disinfectant, viruses that may be on them are killed.

The hands are an important focus of transmission through water, food, blood, respiratory drops, the digestive tract and direct and indirect contact.

-How should you wash your hands?

For an effective wash you have to apply soap in abundance and scrub your palms until you generate a lot of foam. Then this should be passed between the fingers, under the nails and the outer side of the hands.

Then you have to rub your fingertips several times against your palms, including your thumbs. Finally, you have to rub the wrists with the opposite hand and rinse with plenty of water. The wash should last at least 20 seconds.

-What are the key moments for hand hygiene?

It is essential to wash your hands after sneezing or coughing; after being in contact with an infected person; before, during and after cooking; before eating; after going to the bathroom; after touching an animal; upon arrival at the house and after touching elevator buttons, door handles and stair rails, among other moments.

97. Alcohol and antibacterial

-How can we wash our hands if there is no water available?

In these cases, a 75% alcohol-based hand sanitizer can be used, which is effective in inactivating the virus.

-How do you apply the hand sanitizer gel?

It is applied to the palm of one hand and rubs across the entire surface of both hands and fingers until it has dried. This process should take at least 20 seconds.

-Is 75% alcohol also effective for disinfecting surfaces and objects?

Yes. 75% alcohol, chloroform, formaldehyde, disinfectants containing chlorine, peracetic acid, and ultraviolet rays can inactivate the virus, so cleaning surfaces and objects with alcohol can prevent infection.

-Does spraying the body with alcohol or chlorine kill the virus?

No. This is useless since the virus is found inside the body. Spraying alcohol or chlorine can damage clothing and mucous membranes of the eyes and mouth, making it dangerous.

Its use is only effective to disinfect surfaces and objects.

-Does rinsing your nose regularly with saline help prevent infection with COVID-19?

No. There is no evidence to suggest that this practice protects against infection.

98. Lifestyle, exercise and mental health

-What lifestyle is recommended during the pandemic?

Right now it is important to eat well, exercise regularly and get adequate rest a minimum of 7 hours per day.

On the other hand, it is necessary to maintain good hygiene and ventilate the rooms frequently.

Lastly, it is recommended not to overwork, do relaxing and recreational activities and avoid crowded places.

-Why is it important to exercise regularly?

Practicing physical activity helps improve general health, quality of life and sleep. It also allows you to maintain an adequate weight, collaborates in stress management and reduces the chances of contracting certain diseases, such as type 2 diabetes, cardiovascular problems, obesity, osteoporosis, joint pain, and breast and colon cancer.

-What exercise routine is recommended during the pandemic?

During this time a comprehensive and constant program is recommended in which each part of the body is exercised, increasing the intensity progressively.

If it is not possible to go outside or go to a gym due to quarantine, it is recommended to search the internet for training routines to do at home.

-What can we do to prepare ourselves mentally to face the pandemic?

During this stage it is understandable to feel a little anxiety and fear. This is natural and you should not feel guilty about experiencing these emotions.

On the contrary, you have to find a way to let off steam, distract yourself and relieve anxiety.

The practice of physical activity on a regular basis; the use of relaxation techniques such as meditation, yoga, acupuncture or massage; spend more time with family and friends; and engaging in rewarding activities, such as reading, listening to music, drawing, or learning to play a musical instrument, can help manage stress.

In case fear and anxiety become unbearable, seek professional support.

99. Ventilation of houses and rooms

-Why is it important to ventilate the house?

Home and workplace environments are often closed, especially during winter and low temperature days. This causes the air in the rooms to be polluted quickly, due to confinement and indoor activities such as cooking.

-How much should a space be ventilated?

If the outside air is good, it is recommended to ventilate at least three times a day, in the morning, afternoon and evening. Ventilation should be maintained for at least 15 to 30 minutes.

100. Care in quarantine

-What special care must be followed during quarantine?

During quarantine, avoid going outside and maintain face-to-face contact with other people as much as possible.

In addition, preventive care must be followed to the maximum, related to frequent hand washing and disinfection of surfaces and objects.

On the other hand, you must maintain good personal and household hygiene, and cover your nose and mouth with a disposable tissue when coughing or sneezing.

101. Homes for the elderly and disabled

-*What special care must be followed in nursing homes and disabled?*

In these centers, outdoor activities, the entry of new residents and visits by family and friends should be restricted to reduce the risks of contagion.

On the other hand, the place must take extreme measures of hygiene, disinfection and personal and environmental protection.

In addition, workers must be trained on how to prevent, control, and identify cases of COVID-19. These, in turn, must educate and promote care among residents.

If an infected is detected, it should be isolated and quarantined immediately to avoid transmission to others.

102. Markets and supermarkets

-*What care must be taken in markets and supermarkets to avoid contagion?*

In these cases, it is advisable to plan your purchases in advance and purchase everything at once so that you do not have to go to the same place several times.

Within the premises, it is recommended to avoid the busiest hours and always maintain a safety distance of two meters with other clients.

It is important not to talk about food, much less cough or sneeze on it.

In addition, it is advisable to bring your own shopping bags to avoid using the supermarket carts and baskets, and pay by card to avoid having to touch bills and coins.

103. Restaurants and dining rooms

-What care should be taken in restaurants and dining rooms?

In these spaces it is advisable to eat outside the usual hours to avoid the crowds.

If you are accompanied, during food you should avoid contact and face-to-face conversation. Also the desktop, to reduce the stay in the place as much as possible.

On the other hand, it is advisable to use personal or disposable plates, glasses and cutlery that are not shared with others. Also, you have to wash your hands before and after eating.

Personnel working in restaurants and canteens should wear masks and gloves along with regular protective equipment. In turn, on a daily basis, they should take their temperature and look for symptoms related to the virus, such as cough, diarrhea or breathing problems to avoid affecting food security.

Finally, in these places, hygiene, cleaning and disinfection measures must also be extreme.

104. Cinemas and theaters

-What care should be taken in cinemas and theaters?

During the pandemic, it is recommended to avoid visits to crowded and poorly ventilated places such as cinemas and theaters.

If necessary, wear a face mask and keep as much distance as possible from the rest of the spectators.

On the other hand, the organizers of these spaces must guarantee the daily hygiene, ventilation and sterilization of the rooms.

105. Lifts and stairs

-What care must be taken in elevators and stairs?

The elevator should be taken with as few people as possible and wearing a protective mask. The ideal is to travel one by one and, if it is full, it is best to wait for the next one.

Preferably, the use of stairs is recommended to go from one floor to another.

Returning to the elevator, the buttons must be pressed with a disposable tissue and the doors must be kept open longer to increase ventilation. In addition, its interior must be cleaned and disinfected regularly.

As for the stairs, you have to respect the distance with other people and you don't have to touch the railings or the handrails, or do it with disposable gloves.

106. Public and private transportation

-What care must be taken in transportation?

In public transport a protective mask must be used. In addition, in the case of having to wait for the arrival of the bus or the subway, you should avoid sitting on the benches and keeping a safe distance from other people.

If the vehicle arrives and is full, it is recommended to wait for the next one. When paying, preferably you must use prepaid cards or carry the exact change, so you do not have to exchange money with the collector.

Inside the bus, if possible, sit on empty benches with no people next to you. In turn, before holding on to the safety rails, it is advisable to clean your hands with gel alcohol.

Once the trip is over, you have to wash your hands again with soap and water.

107. Flights and airports

-What care should be taken on flights and airports?

Ideally, avoid traveling during the pandemic.

In case you have to do it, it is recommended to check in online before going to the airport and download the boarding pass on your cell phone to avoid handling paperwork, contact with other people and waste of time.

On the other hand, it is advisable to avoid using the airport and airplane toilets.

Once in the seat, it is recommended to disinfect the belts, armrests, reclining tables and touch screen with gel alcohol and to activate the vents.

108. Ports and cruises

-What care should be taken in ports and cruise ships?

Ideally, avoid taking cruises during the pandemic.

If you must, stay in your cabin as long as possible. In common places, keep a distance of more than two meters with other passengers. In the dining room use your own or disposable plates and cutlery. Wash your hands frequently and follow general advice to prevent the virus.

109. Schools and universities

-What care should be taken in schools and universities?

In these establishments, students and teachers must be made aware of prevention, control and safety measures through talks and training.

In addition, action protocols must be established to detect possible cases and ensure that those infected enter into quarantine. This may include daily examination of students and teachers for symptoms.

On the other hand, cleaning staff should increase hygiene, ventilation and disinfection of classrooms and items for public use.

Group meetings and activities should also be discouraged. In classrooms, students must sit separately, maintaining an adequate distance from each other.

Finally, times should be organized in gyms, libraries, laboratories and dining rooms so that there are as few people as possible at one time.

Part X. Summary of facts and clinical controversies

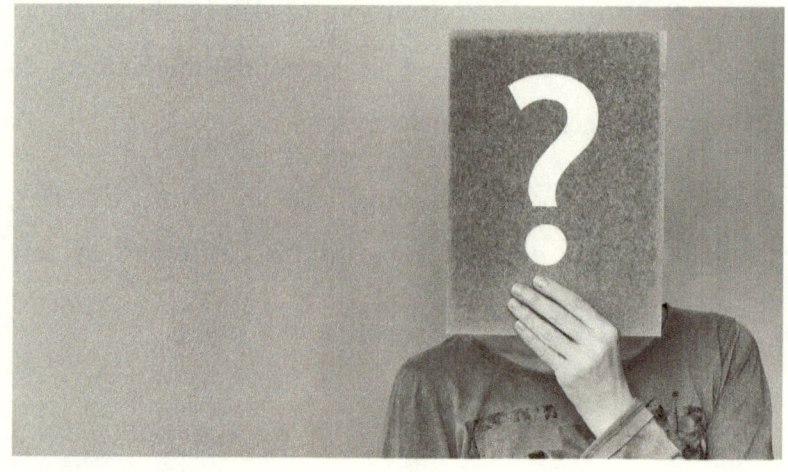

In this last part of the book we will dedicate you to answer some questions, as well as clarify doubts and myths about prevention measures, diagnosis, symptoms, complications, immunity, and treatments.

Handwashing with soap, sodium hypochlorite, and antiseptic alcohol removes the virus.

True. Hand washing is very important because when it is done with soap and water or using an alcohol-based disinfectant, viruses that may be on them are killed.

Quarantine, social distance and the use of masks will avoid infecting us.

True. These measures serve to reduce the potential for disease transmission. If applied correctly and on a large scale, social distance, quarantine and the use of masks break or decrease the chain of contagion. This helps protect the vulnerable public and reduces the burden of care in hospitals, avoiding the collapse of the health system.

People who have the virus without symptoms can transmit it.

True. It is proven that asymptomatic patients can transmit the disease. That is why it is important that even without showing signs they comply with the quarantine.

It is a simple flu that attacks older people with low defenses.

False. This virus is 30 times more lethal than the common flu and almost twice as contagious. It also attacks people of all ages.

Only older people and people with previous medical conditions get complicated and die.

False. While it is true that older people and those with previous medical conditions present much greater risks, there have also been cases of patients who did not have previous health problems who suffered complications. So it is important that we all take care of ourselves.

Healthy children and youth are less susceptible to the virus.

True. Preliminary research shows that healthy children and youth are less susceptible.

There is a difference between protective inflammatory and hyperinflammatory response.

True. When an attack by a bacteria or virus occurs, the immune system can activate a protective inflammatory response as a defense mechanism. In these cases the damaged tissue releases chemicals that cause inflammation. This helps isolate the foreign substance and attracts white blood cells to destroy it.

However, sometimes this response can be severe and hyperinflammatory. The chemicals that the same organism releases into the blood flow can cause changes that damage multiple body systems and worsen the condition.

One of the most serious complications is "cytokine storm and hemophagocytic lymphohistiocytosis."

True. Cytokine storm is a serious immune reaction in which too many cytokines are released into the blood by the body too quickly. These proteins play an important role in immune responses, but can be harmful when produced in large quantities.

In cases of COVID-19, some patients respond to the virus with a cytokine storm, exacerbating their condition by causing failure of multiple organs.

Hemophagocytic lymphohistiocytosis, meanwhile, is a rare disorder in which histiocytes and lymphocytes (types of white blood cells) accumulate in the organs and destroy other blood cells. The trigger factor can be an infection -like COVID-19- and mainly affects people who have immunity deficiencies, autoimmune disorders or cancer.

The virus enters the body's cells through the ECA-II receptor.

True. The renin-angiotensin-aldosterone axis is a hormonal system that regulates blood pressure, body extracellular volume, and the balance of sodium and potassium in the body.

Renin is secreted by the cells of the juxtaglomerular apparatus of the kidney. It catalyzes the movement of angiotensinogen, a glycoprotein secreted in the liver, into angiotensin I. In turn, it is converted to angiotensin II by the action of the enzyme known as ACE-2 or ACE-2 in the lungs and other tissues, and organs.

One of the ways the new virus enters the body's cells is by using the enzyme ACE-2 or ECA-2 as a receptor.

Stopping treatments for hypertension, diabetes and rheumatoid arthritis helps against the virus.

False. These patients must continue with their treatments and intensify controls and preventive measures. In no case should they suspend their medications or self-medicate without the supervision of a professional. Adherence to treatment is even more important in these times.

There is currently no evidence to support discontinuation of these drugs, including angiotensin-converting enzyme ACE inhibitors and angiotensin receptor blockers (ARBs), used for example to treat hypertension.

Loss of smell and taste among the first symptoms.

True in some cases. Some patients with COVID-19 have reported difficulties in detecting taste and odors. Although at the moment the cause for which this occurs is not known, it is being investigated.

These people reported a sudden loss of their senses of taste and smell, even without experiencing the most common symptoms of the disease, such as fever, cough, sore throat, or difficulty breathing. These signs appear to appear early in the infection, so they may help detect your infection early.

There are helpful alarm signs for isolated minor patients in your home to avoid dying at home.

True. These patients should control fever and contact a doctor in cases where it is above 38 degrees, or when they have difficulty breathing, constant chest pain or pressure, changes in mental state, confusion, trouble waking up or a bluish tint to the lips or face.

There are different courses in the pathogenesis, clinic and treatment between the phases of COVID-19

True. In cases of mild illness, the patients do not have symptoms or they are very mild - a little cough, fever below 38 degrees, nasal congestion, general malaise. These patients do not require hospitalization and can recover and quarantine at home.

In cases of severe disease, patients have a respiratory rate of more than 30 breaths per minute; a blood oxygen saturation of less than 93%; a Kirby or PaO2 / FiO2 ratio less than 300; and pulmonary infiltrates greater than 50% in 24-48 hours.

When the oxygen saturation value is less than 90%, supplemental oxygen therapy is applied, which may include a nasal catheter, an oxygen mask, high-flow transnasal oxygen therapy, and non-invasive or invasive mechanical ventilation, among other possibilities.

If acute hypoxemic respiratory failure does not respond to conventional treatment, a high-flow nasal cannula (HFNC) and non-invasive positive pressure ventilation (NIPPV) can be used.

In severe cases, patients present respiratory failure with the need for mechanical ventilation or septic shock. Treatment includes oxygen therapy, fluid replacement, antibacterial treatments, corticosteroids, and tests with antivirals that are being studied.

All pneumonias require X-rays, ultrasounds, and CT scans.

False. However, these studies provide interesting indicators to take into account to speed up the diagnosis, start treatment and isolate patients when necessary, so its use is recommended.

The RT-PCR molecular diagnostic test and the rapid diagnostic tests for SARS-CoV2 are different.

True. The PCR test seeks to detect the presence of a molecule of ribonucleic acid (RNA), the genetic material of the virus. It has the advantage that it is very specific, since it allows to differentiate between two very similar pathogens.

In addition, this test is very effective, because it covers the virus in the early stages of infection. Its disadvantage is that the results take between 4 hours and two days.

Rapid tests, meanwhile, use blood samples to detect antibodies produced against the disease, or respiratory samples to look for virus proteins.

Unlike PCR, these tests are useful from the fifth day of infection. They also have the disadvantage that they are not as effective and specific. As a point in favor, they allow you to obtain the results in just 15 minutes.

Procalcitonin as a marker of bacterial infection.

True. The level of procalcitonin (a protein that is produced in the body in some cases) in the blood is usually normal at the beginning of the disease but increases in patients who require intensive care. Therefore, it is recommended to perform tests to monitor this indicator regularly, since it may indicate a secondary complication of bacterial infection.

The disease can cause extrapulmonary symptoms and multi-organ failure.

True. When the virus begins to spread, it can cause various symptoms throughout the body. It is unclear whether this occurs as a consequence of a direct viral manifestation or due to the inflammatory response.

Some common signs are mental confusion, cognitive decline, and seizures in the central nervous system; renal and adrenal insufficiency; myocarditis in the heart; and systemic vasculitis.

In the case of multi-organ failure it is generally caused by the cytokine storm.

There are reliable predictors of severity or mortality that allow taking advanced medical actions.

True. Patients with severe pneumonia, dyspnea, and hypoxemia that affect more than 50% of the lung in 24-48 hours require urgent treatment to prevent progression to sepsis, septic shock, and multiple organ dysfunction syndrome.

In turn, within these predictors are the respiratory rate of more than 30 breaths per minute; blood oxygen saturation less than 93%; a Kirby or PaO2 / FiO2 ratio less than 300; and pulmonary infiltrates greater than 50 percent in 24-48 hours.

Oseltamivir and other antivirals may be treatments.

False. At the moment there is no proven antiviral therapy that works against this virus. However, some drugs are being used with the compassionate use procedure, reserved for not-yet-approved drugs used in patients who have no other therapeutic option.

Oseltamivir is an antiviral that is used to treat some types of influenza infection (another type of virus that causes flu-like syndrome) and is part of the drugs that are being tested against COVID-19. It is recommended for cases of moderate illness.

Ivermectin or nitazoxanide are medicines to treat the disease.

False. Ivermectin is an anthelmintic medicine indicated for the treatment of parasitoses such as strongyloidiasis, onchocerciasis and scabies. It has been used to combat HIV, dengue, the flu, Zikay, among other ailments.

Nitazoxanide is an antiparasitic that is used to treat diarrhea caused by the protozoan cryptosporidium or giardia. Both drugs are under study against COVID-19.

The treatment for hospitalized patients is azithromycin, chloroquine, and hydroxychloroquine.

Partially true. Chloroquine and hydroxychloroquine are two antimalarials that are also used to treat autoimmune diseases such as lupus and some types of arthritis. Azithromycin, meanwhile, is an antibiotic.

The use of these associated drugs against COVID-19 is being studied. Its implementation is recommended in cases where there are evident risk factors for disease progression.

Among the adverse reactions of chloroquine, dizziness, headache, nausea, vomiting, diarrhea, different types of skin rashes and cardiac arrest have been identified.

Using fresh plasma or immunoglobulins from recovered patients can help treat other patients and prevent infections.

In study. This treatment involves removing blood plasma from people who have recovered from the disease to treat critically ill patients.

This plasma - which is administered through a transfusion - contains antibodies capable of attacking the virus and helping patients to recover faster.

Interferon, monoclonal antibodies, and intravenous immunoglobulins are treatments.

In study. Interferon is a molecule produced by the body itself to fight viral infections and to help regulate inflammation. Its use in patients with COVID-19 is recommended for critical cases.

Monoclonal antibodies are proteins used by the immune system to identify and neutralize foreign objects, such as bacteria and viruses. Its use could block the ability of the new coronavirus to penetrate cells.

Intravenous immunoglobulin, for its part, is a substance that is made with antibodies that are extracted from the blood of healthy donors. An early dose could improve the prognosis of critically ill patients with COVID-19.

Troponins and other enzymes indicate endothelial damage, heart damage, and acute myocardial infarction.

True. Elevated troponins are a marker of myocardial damage. In turn, the cardiac marker test measures the release in the blood of various enzymes that help diagnose a heart attack.

Heart failure occurs when the heart muscle does not pump blood properly. Certain conditions, such as narrowed arteries or high blood pressure, progressively leave the heart too weak or stiff to fill and pump effectively.

Acute myocardial infarction, also known as heart attack, occurs as a consequence of insufficient blood supply to the heart and the consequent lack of oxygen.

Health professionals must protect themselves more from cardiorespiratory arrest.

True. Cardiorespiratory arrest involves the sudden and unexpected cessation of blood circulation and spontaneous breathing. This generates a lack of oxygen to the vital organs, especially damaging the brain. When it stops receiving oxygen for 6-8 minutes, the death of its cells occurs, producing an irreversible situation.

In resuscitation procedures, medical personnel should use N95 masks, face shields, latex gloves, waterproof insulation clothing, protective clothing, and respirator, if necessary, as protective measures.

In unemployment improve airway with: Ambu, laryngeal masks and endotracheal intubation.

True. To improve the airway area of patients who are not breathing or who are having trouble breathing on their own, a manual resuscitator known as Ambu can be used. It is a self-expanding bag mask that provides positive pressure ventilation.

Other options are to put on a laryngeal mask or perform an endotracheal intubation. In the latter case, a probe is placed in the windpipe through the mouth or nose.

In cardiac resuscitation the sequence is: defibrillation, cardiac massage technique in pronation, medication.

It depends on the cause of the cardiac arrest. In the event of cardiac arrest, an immediate CPR cardiopulmonary resuscitation procedure must be performed. Mouth-to-mouth breathing is combined with chest compressions, to supply oxygen to the lungs and keep blood circulating until breathing and heart palpitations can be restored.

Advanced care continues with defibrillation, in which a device is used to give an electrical shock to the heart. This causes it to stop momentarily and then resume its normal rhythm.

Finally, certain antiarrhythmic medications may also be necessary to treat the emergency or for long-term therapy.

To study cardiac damage, an echocardiogram, interventional coronary angiography, and thrombolysis are performed.

True. Echocardiography is a test that creates images of the heart and helps diagnose defects in the organ.

For its part, coronary angiography is a procedure in which a catheter is inserted into an artery in the arm or groin, which is carefully brought to the heart, allowing the obstruction of blood flow to be detected.

Thrombolysis, meanwhile, is a process in which blood clots break down using medications.

It helps the immunomodulatory effect of statins, propolis, homeopathic drops and levamisole.

In study. Statins are drugs that lower cholesterol and certain fats in the blood, which helps reduce cardiovascular disease. They also have an immunomodulatory and anti-inflammatory effect. Evidence of their role in patients with COVID19 is scarce.

Propolis is a material produced by bees that is used to treat swelling and sores inside the mouth. Its use could help strengthen the immune system and function as a natural antiviral.

As for homeopathic drops, there is currently no scientific evidence that their use increases defenses against viral diseases and respiratory infections.

Levamisole, meanwhile, is an anthelmintic and immunomodulatory medication. At the moment, there is also no certainty that it is effective in preventing or treating COVID-19.

Improves defenses: vitamin D, B-complex vitamin serums and vitamin C overdose

False. There is no scientific evidence that these vitamins are effective in preventing COVID-19 infection. Furthermore, taking and injecting vitamin C, vitamin supplements and other preparations do not have an immediate effect. Its use has to be long-term, in a correct way and combined with a healthy lifestyle to be effective.

Anyway, to improve the functioning of the immune system it is best to follow a balanced diet, exercise moderately and maintain a good state of mental health.

For its part, vitamin D supplementation could help prevent acute respiratory infections.

Effective vaccines may be available in less than 2 years.

True. It is estimated that its development can take between 6 months and a year and a half. The deadlines are generally much longer, but it is possible that in this global crisis situation there will be more flexibility for international regulatory bodies to approve it.

It affects pregnancy, childbirth and the newborn.

Not checked. Unlike other infectious diseases, pregnant women with COVID-19 do not appear to develop a more severe clinical picture than the general population. There is also no evidence that the disease increases the risk of miscarriage.

Furthermore, the first studies indicate that there is no vertical transmission before, during and after childbirth from infected mothers to offspring.

It will harm children psychomotor and intellectual development.

False. COVID-19 affects children in a very small proportion compared to adults. In addition, in these few cases the disease is usually very mild and does not usually leave sequelae.

Recovered patients may leave isolation and the use of masks.

True. To be discharged, these patients must be stable and fever free, and the lung images must show significant improvement with no signs of organ dysfunction.

Furthermore, breathing and speech must be normalized and the person must be in clear consciousness for at least 3 days. Finally, they must have two consecutive negative results performed on different days of the PCR test.

Recovered patients are immune to SARS-Cov2.

In study. It is still too early to give an answer. At the moment, there are no determining scientific data on the duration of the protective immune antibodies generated in patients who had the disease and were cured. However, these patients may be protected from future infections.

Most people who became infected with SARS developed long-term immunity, ranging from eight to ten years. In the case of MERS it was much shorter. It is estimated that immunity against COVID-19 could be at least 1 or 2 years old, although at the moment there are no concrete data.

Leaves functional sequelae or pulmonary fibrosis in recovered patients

In study. However, although it is still too premature to draw conclusions because the disease is very recent, cases have been detected in which the lung is left with some type of fibrosis.

Like this also depends on what was the state of the organ before the disease.

Volume 2

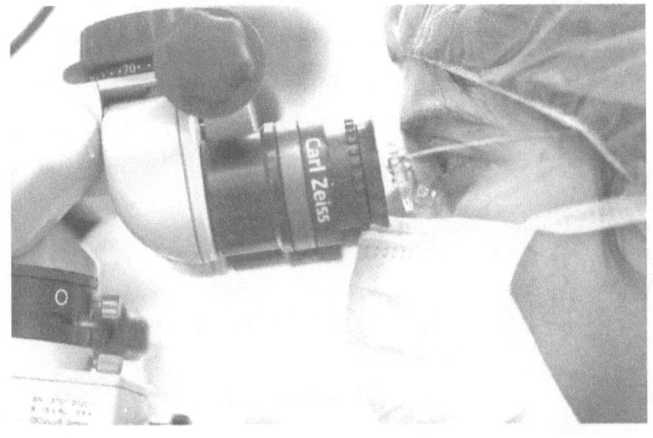

*Aimed at health professionals, to enrich their knowledge
regarding SARS-CoV-2 and pathology COVID-19*

Novel-coronavirus Guide

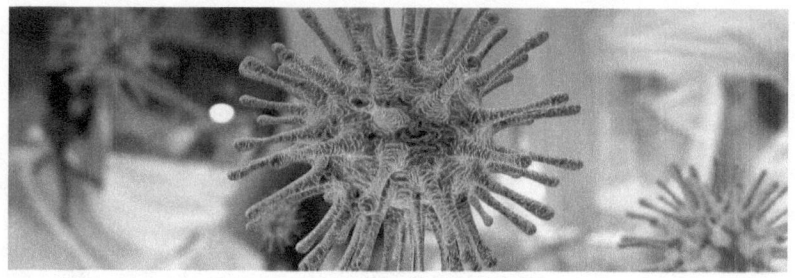

Dr. Mario Vega Carbó

Endocrinologist

Edition 2021

-Volume N° 2-

Background and timeline of the pandemic

The new coronavirus COVID-19 first appeared in Wuhan City, Hubei Province of China in early December 2019.

In just one month, the number of cases grew exponentially and just 3 months later it is already a global pandemic.

The key dates of this pandemic are described below:

On December 8, 2019, seven cases of a strange disease that caused symptoms similar to pneumonia were reported in Wuhan, Hubei province, China.

On December 21 of that year, the Chinese Center for Disease Control identified a first group of 15 patients affected by pneumonia of unknown cause.

On December 30, 2019, the genetic sequencing of the pathogen in one patient indicated the presence, not yet fully confirmed, of a coronavirus related to Severe Acute Respiratory Syndrome (SARS).

In addition, the majority of the ill patients were found to be workers or customers of the Wuhan Wholesale Seafood Market, of which seven were in critical condition.

On December 31, 2019, an urgent notice of the presence of pneumonia of unknown cause was issued to the Wuhan Municipal Health Center. At this time there are already dozens of patients affected in hospitals in this city.

For its part, in January the origin of this disease was discovered and cases began to appear outside of China. This month marked the beginning of the worldwide expansion of the new coronavirus.

On January 9, 2020, "Patient Zero" died, a 61-year-old man who claimed to have become ill after visiting the Wuhan Seafood Market.

That same day, Chinese health authorities notified the World Health Organization (WHO) that they have identified a new type of coronavirus, called 2019-nCoV, as causing the pneumonia outbreak in Wuhan.

On January 13, the WHO reported the first case of COVID-19 outside of China, in this case in Thailand. The victim was a 61-year-old Chinese woman who had flown to Bangkok five days earlier.

On January 16, Japan reported its first case to a resident of Kanagawa Prefecture.

On January 20, South Korea informed the WHO that it had confirmed a first case. Simultaneously, Chinese researchers identified three different strains of the 2019-nCoV earlier that day, confirming that the original coronavirus that appeared in Wuhan had mutated.

While the announcement of this discovery was made, the United States confirmed the appearance of the first case in that country, in the state of Washington.

Singapore reported its first case **on January 23**, in a person who came from Wuhan, as did Taiwan and Vietnam.

On January 23, the Chinese government ordered a total quarantine for the 11 million inhabitants of Wuhan, as well as the cancellation of flights and train departures to and from this city.

The operation of trains, buses and ferries in the entire metropolitan area of this city was also suspended.

By this date, 17 people had already died in China and another 580 had been infected outside of this country.

On January 24, the first report of COVID-19 was recorded in Europe, in two French who arrived in Paris by flight from Wuhan, while China reported that it already had 830 infected in its continental territory.

For its part, **on January 25** Australia reported that 3 nationals who arrived from Wuhan were diagnosed with COVID-19.

That same day, Canada reported its first case in the city of Toronto, also in a tourist who had returned from Wuhan.

On January 27, Germany reported its first case to a national from the Bayern region who returned from Shanghai, China.

On January 29, COVID-19 reached the Persian Gulf, when the United Arab Emirates informed the WHO that it had 4 confirmed cases of this virus, all in people who were in Wuhan, China.

On January 30, the WHO reported that COVID-19 was present in all provinces of mainland China, as well as in several countries in Europe, North and South America.

On this date the WHO declared a state of global health emergency due to the COVID-19 outbreak, which had already killed 170 people in China and sickened 7,711 people.

At that time, China had ordered the complete closure of Wuhan and the cessation of all non-essential activities so that the population would remain isolated and reduce person-to-person contagion.

That same day, Italy reported its first two cases, but no special measure was issued to prevent the spread of the contagion, except for restrictions on travelers from China.

The month of February marked the beginning of the rapid spread of COVID-19 in Europe, Latin America and Europe, where several countries had to apply extreme measures of social isolation and border closures to try to stop the epidemic.

The date of **February 28** stands out, when the first two cases were reported in Latin America, in 2 Mexicans who had visited Italy. Immediately Chile, Colombia and Brazil cases were reported.

The month of March marks the declaration of a global pandemic of COVID-19 by the World Health Organization and the exponential increase in confirmed cases on all continents except Africa.

From March 5 to 6, the appearance of COVID-19 was reported in Central and South America, in this case in Argentina, Peru, Colombia and Costa Rica.

As of March 7, more than 90 countries were facing the presence of COVID-19 and 102,000 infected people had been registered and nearly 3,500 deaths. That day Paraguay reported its first case of coronavirus.

On March 9 Germany reports that it has 1,100 cases of COVID-19 and the first 2 deaths occur in that country.

On March 12, the WHO reports that worldwide there are 126,100 infected with COVID-19 and 4,600 deaths.

On March 14, the WHO reports that Europe is the new epicenter of the COVID-19 epidemic and the United States declares a state of national health emergency. For this day, the infected in the world exceed 145,300 people and there are 5,500 deaths.

In contrast, the WHO reported that 71,600 people had recovered, mostly in China.

On March 16 the situation in Europe forces the European Union to close internal borders. Portugal reports the first death from this coronavirus.

On March 18, Spain reaches 11,178 infected and 491 deceased. While worldwide, 218,000 are reported infected, 8,809 deceased and 84,000 people recovered.

Just a day later, Italy reached 3,405 deaths, surpassing China, which had 3,252 registered. Globally, the number of infected rises to 244,000, with 10,000 deaths and 86,000 recoveries.

On March 25, Spain exceeded the number of deaths in China, with 3,434 deaths, of which 738 deaths had occurred in the last 24 hours.

On March 27, Spain registers 769 deaths in just 24 hours. In the world, those infected are over 500,000 people, of whom 88,000 correspond to the United States. This puts the US above China and Italy in number of infections.

On March 30, Spain surpassed China in number of positive cases, and worldwide more than 700 thousand people were infected throughout the planet.

To this are added more than 30 thousand deaths from complications related to this disease.

Part I. Defenses, airways and viruses

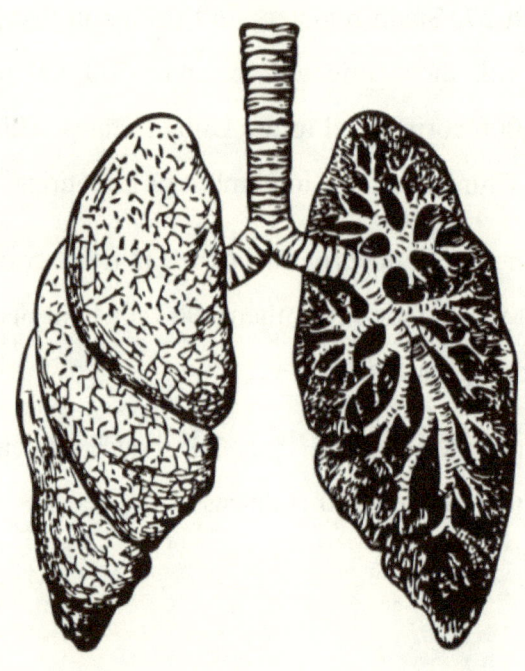

The human body has an immune system to protect itself from infections and external pathogens.

This system is made up of a variety of blood cells, called white blood cells or lymphocytes, specially adapted to detect and destroy microorganisms outside the body.

Different body structures such as the spleen and the bone marrow participate in the formation of these cells.

In addition, the body has structures that help filter and remove toxins and pathogens from the blood flow. Lymph nodes are the main structures of this type.

1. Types of immunity

The term immunity comes from the Latin immunis, which means "free of charge". This term refers to the general ability of an organism or host to resist a given infection or disease.

At the beginning of the 20th century, the concepts of "antibody" were defined to refer to the proteins produced by the cells of the immune system that participate in humoral immunity and "antigens" for substances that bind to the antibodies or stimulate their production.

Defense against an infectious agent is based on a combination of the early organic response related to innate immunity and the subsequent response arising from the adaptive immunity that the body has developed.

As innate immunity, also called natural, describes the mechanisms that the body has to protect itself from infections, before they appear.

These mechanisms are the body's first line of defense against infection. They include chemical and physical barriers, phagocytic cells, natural cytotoxic cells, and blood proteins.

For its part, adaptive immunity, also called acquired, is one that the body develops by stimulation after being exposed to pathogens. In this case, immunity is selective and specific for each type of infectious agent. The main culprits for this adaptive immunity are lymphocytes.

There are two types of adaptive immunity, such as humoral immunity and cellular immunity.

2. Humoral and cellular immunity

Cellular immunity is based on the defense of the organism through the activation of cellular called T lymphocytes, mainly in the presence of intracellular microorganisms.

For its part, humoral immunity is based on the defense of the organism through the action of macromolecules called antibodies. In this case, they are generally activated to attack infections by extracellular microorganisms and the toxins they produce.

This defense mechanism in turn has the ability to recall the fought infection, through memory B lymphocytes. In this way, if the infection reappears, the body's defenses will be activated faster and more efficiently to fight it.

However, it cannot be said that they are two totally separate forms of immunity, since the cells and physiological processes that participate in both types of response are closely related.

3. Active and passive immunity

Another form of resistance to infection is active immunity, in which the body's immune system is motivated to react when exposed to an antigen or specific immunogenic structure.

For its part, passive immunity consists of that which is acquired by the individual by external transfer. This means that it is an immunity acquired without having been exposed to the antigen corresponding to a certain infection, as is the case of the immunity that the mother transfers to the fetus or that acquired after being treated against rabies or tetanus.

4. Defense against biological agents

Every living organism has mechanisms to protect itself from the damaging action of biological agents. These can be nonspecific or specific mechanisms.

The nonspecific mechanisms react to any pathogen or foreign substance that enters the organism, destroying them as soon as possible. Non-specific mechanisms include natural barriers, the microflora, and the inflammatory response or non-specific cellular response.

Natural barriers, also called primary barriers, are made up of animal skin and plant epidermis, as well as mucous secretions. Its function is to block the entry of pathogens into the body through a physical or mechanical barrier.

The skin acts as a wall against external agents, thanks to its thickness, waterproof capacity, and slight acidity due to the release of fatty acids in the sebaceous glands. Vaginal secretions, nasal mucus and stomach mucosa also protect against the entry of bacteria into the body, thanks to its bactericidal enzymes. Mucus from the nose and airways helps trap and expel foreign substances and bacteria from the lungs through sneezing and coughing.

As for microflora, they are commensal strains of bacteria that form symbiosis with the human and animal bodies and protect them against foreign bacteria by competing with them for nutrients and releasing substances that affect their development. The skin and intestine are covered by thousands of such symbiotic microorganisms.

For its part, the inflammatory response or non-specific cellular response, consists of a reaction of the cells to protect themselves from pathogens, in many cases producing substances such as interferons, which prevent viruses from starting their multiplication process.

The production of histamines and other substances produce a dilation of the blood vessels in the affected area and therefore, an inflammation is generated.

5. Anatomy of the airways

From the anatomical point of view, the human respiratory system is made up of the following structures:

Upper respiratory tract.

Lower respiratory tract.

Diaphragmatic muscles and accessories.

The upper airways are made up of the nose and pharynx. The pharynx in turn communicates with the lower airways, made up of the bronchi and bronchioles located within the lungs.

The lungs in turn are made up of millions of structures called alveoli, where the exchange of CO_2 and O_2 takes place between the atmosphere and the body. In turn, the lungs and lower airways are located inside the thorax, surrounded by the ribs.

The entry and exit of air from the lungs, which we know as the action of breathing, is caused by the regular movement of the diaphragm, a dome-like set of muscles located below the lungs. By raising and lowering and lowering the diaphragm, it causes the lungs to fill or empty with air by mechanical effect.

6. Barriers, mucosa and respiratory epithelium

As we said before, the body has natural barriers to protect itself from the entry of bacteria, viruses and dangerous substances. In the case of the lungs, the nasal mucosa and the respiratory epithelium are the main protective structures.

The respiratory epithelium is itself a ciliated epithelium, that is, it has thousands of small hairs or beards and which covers the entire respiratory tract. The movement of their beards or cilia, combined with the mucus that is continuously secreted, helps to expel dead bacteria, dust and pathogens that may be inside them from the lungs. In severe cases, the cough mechanism is activated to help expel phlegm or excessive mucus.

The nasal mucosa in turn produces a large amount of mucus and is the first physical barrier against the entry of foreign particles and bacteria into the lungs. Upon detecting the presence of these, an allergic reaction occurs characterized by increased mucus and sneezing, which help to expel bacteria from the upper respiratory tract.

7. Acute and respiratory infections

Various acute diseases of the respiratory system caused by viruses and bacteria that appear suddenly and whose symptoms last less than 15 days are grouped under the term Acute Respiratory Infection (ARI).

ARF is the most frequent type of respiratory disease on the planet, and its variants include from mild colds to severe colds and pneumonia, among others.

Viruses are the most common cause of respiratory infections and in addition to affecting the lungs and bronchi, they can also present problems at the ear level (otitis) and sinuses (sinusitis).

However, there are very dangerous bacterial diseases, such as tuberculosis caused by the Koch Bacillus, which can cause the death of the patient, both due to damage to his respiratory system and other organs.

Generally speaking, the most common respiratory infections are the common cold, pharyngitis, and rhinosinusitis. The common cold is characterized by nasal congestion, increased runny nose, sneezing and coughing, headache, and malaise.

Pharyngitis is notable for a sore throat, often accompanied by symptoms of the common cold and white plaques or painful lumps in the throat and tonsils. Its cause may be viral or bacterial.

For its part, rhinosinusitis is an infection that affects the mucosa of the paranasal sinuses and nose. Its symptoms include facial pain, nasal congestion, fever, and general discomfort. It can be caused by a virus or bacteria.

8. Most common respiratory viruses

Data from the World Health Organization indicate that there are more than 150 viruses in the world that can cause respiratory diseases of some kind.

However, the most common are rhinoviruses, responsible for the common cold, as well as Influenza virus, Parainfluenza, Adenovirus, and Respiratory Syncytial Virus (RSV).

The Influenza Virus causes what we know as the flu, a highly contagious respiratory disease, with an incubation period of 1 to 3 days. There are two types of influenza viruses, A and B, that mutate periodically and therefore the majority of the population is vulnerable to the new strains that appear. Its symptoms appear suddenly, with fever, chills, muscle and headaches and high fever, as well as abundant discharge of nasal mucus.

Parainfluenza virus is also very frequent, but it mainly affects the lungs, causing inflammation of the bronchi and bronchioles, as well as some types of pneumonia. Its initial symptoms appear to a cold, with runny nose and fever, but chest pain and shortness of breath also appear.

For its part, the Respiratory Syncytial Virus (RSV) causes lung and respiratory tract infections. It mainly affects young children and older adults and its first symptom is dry cough. Depending on age and physical condition, it can lead to a shortness of breath and a very high fever.

Finally we have Adenoviruses, which cause both intestinal and respiratory infections. It can attack throughout the year, but spikes are usually recorded in winter and early summer. In addition to cold-like symptoms, they cause stomach pain, vomiting, and diarrhea that weaken the patient.

9. Bacterial superinfections

In immunosuppressed patients, such as those affected by AIDS, older adults or patients with serious diseases such as cancer, it may be the case that they present infections caused by more than one type of bacteria at the same time.

A viral infection can also cause a drop in the body's ability to fight bacterial infections, opening doors to moderate to severe lung problems. It is common to find immunosuppressed patients whose lung sample cultures show the simultaneous presence of *S. pneumoniae, M. catarrhalis* and *H. influenzae* bacteria. Therefore, they must undergo broad-spectrum antibiotic treatments, which in many cases can also have side effects on the kidneys and liver of high-risk patients.

10. Upper and lower respiratory complications

The most common upper and lower respiratory complications are bronchitis, sinusitis, laryngitis, and otitis.

Bronchitis is an infection of both bacterial and viral origin, which usually manifests itself after flu in the bronchi, causing their inflammation and reducing the passage of air through them. This causes difficulty in breathing as well as a considerable increase in mucus production by the pulmonary epithelium.

Consequently, there is a cough with very strong phlegm, which can last between 3 and 4 weeks, accompanied by fever, sore throat, diarrhea and upset stomach. If not cured in time, it can lead to fibrosis and permanent damage to the lungs.

For its part, pharyngitis is inflammation of the pharynx or back of the throat, caused by a cold, influenza virus, mononucleosis or strep. It causes pain when swallowing or speaking, itchy and dry throat, inflammation of the tonsils and loss of voice. If not treated properly it can spread to the inner ear and sinuses, causing other bothersome symptoms.

Laryngitis is inflammation of the larynx, the organ where the vocal cords are located. It is characterized by total or partial loss of voice, as well as inflammation of the tonsils. It can be caused by viruses, bacteria, or contaminants. One of its most dangerous complications is epiglottitis, in which the epiglottis becomes inflamed and blocks the passage of air to the lungs.

Finally, we have pneumonia, which is inflammation of the lungs by the action of viruses, bacteria, or fungi. This causes the pulmonary alveoli to fill with fluid and pus, reducing the exchange of carbon dioxide and oxygen between the blood and the air when breathing. Up to 15% of infant deaths in children under 5 years of age worldwide are due to pneumonia. Its symptoms include cough with phlegm and blood, chest pain, high fever, and shortness of breath.

Part II Virology, Coronavirus and COVID-19

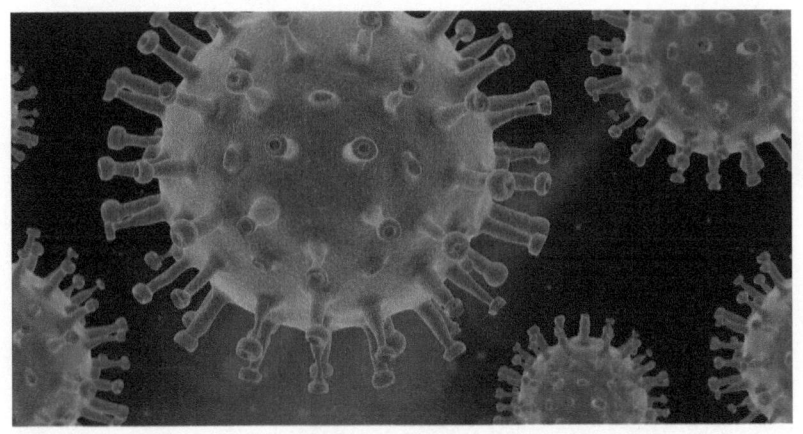

11. Types and characteristics of non-respiratory viruses

There are a large number of viruses that cause organic diseases in humans other than respiratory diseases. One of the most common is gastroenteritis, which can be caused by different types of viruses, such as rotaviruses, noroviruses, astroviruses, and adenoviruses 40 and 41. Most viruses related to gastroenteritis are transmitted orally or by contact with faeces of sick patients.

There are also 5 types of viruses that can cause hepatitis, a disease that affects the liver. Each is identified by a letter (A, B, C, D, and E) that applies to the type of hepatitis it causes.

Cytomegalovirus and Epstein-Barr virus also cause liver problems, as well as Yellow Fever virus.

Other viruses that affect organs other than the lungs are Herpes Simplex virus (HSV), Human Papilloma virus (HPV), and echoviruses. Other very common non-lung diseases caused by viruses are chickenpox, measles, and rubella..

12. Flu and viruses more aggressive to the respiratory tree

Influenza (type A and B), avian influenza A (H5N1 and H7N9) and the Parainfluenza virus (type 1 to 4) are among the most aggressive with the human respiratory system. They are joined by rhinoviruses, respiratory syncytial virus Ay B, adenovirus, and human metapneumovirus.

The best known and most frequent is the Influenza virus, which causes the flu, and whose symptoms are nasal congestion, cough, high fever, vomiting and abdominal pain and diarrhea. It can also be fatal if the individual has special conditions for other diseases, is very old or too young.

Throughout history there have been 6 pandemics caused by the Influenza virus. These are:

Russian Influenza of the year 1889 (H2N2)

Old Hong Kong Influenza of the Year 1900 (H3N8)

Spanish influenza of the year 1918 (H1N1)

1957 Asian Influenza (H2N2)

Hong Kong Influenza 1968 (H3N2)

13. Coronavirus: types, their shape and structure

The name Coronavirus groups together a large and very old family of enveloped RNA viruses. Coronaviruses have a single-stranded, or single stranded, positive sense RNA. This RNA has between 27 to 31 kilonucleotides, making them the largest RNA virus. They also have a phosphorylated protein capsid that binds to the genome forming a ribonucleoprotein helix.

The common ancestor of current coronaviruses has been traced back to around 10,000 years ago, but it is possible that this type of virus existed already for millions of years. Its name "crown" comes from the fact that numerous points protrude from its surface that give it a crown appearance. These tips are used as ligands by fusing with the membranes of invaded cells. There are 12 types of coronavirus are known to affect humans or animals.

However, only 7 of them have the capacity to cause respiratory diseases in humans, ranging from simple colds to very severe pneumonia. Of these seven types of coronaviruses, the following four are related to the common flu:

HcoV-229E.

HcoV-OC43.

HcoV-NL63.

HcoV-HKU1.

On the other hand, the following three types of coronaviruses cause much more serious diseases:

SARS-CoV. Identified in 2002 as causing the Severe Acute Respiratory Syndrome (SARS).

MERS-CoV. Identified in 2012, it is related to Middle East Respiratory Syndrome (MERS).

SARS-CoV-2. This is the most recently discovered and responsible for the 2019 coronavirus disease (COVID-19).

It is noteworthy that the three types that affect humans are zoonotic pathogens, that is, they pass from an animal host to a human host.

14. Classification of coronaviruses

The Coronaviridae family includes two subfamilies and five genera of RNA viruses:

Orthocoronavirinae subfamily (Coronavirus)

Alphacoronavirus genus.

Also called Group 1. It includes varieties such as feline coronavirus, canine coronavirus, and human coronavirus 229E NL63. This genus also includes the coronavirus Miniopterus 1, Miniopterus HKU8, Rhinolophus HKU2, and Scotophilus 512, as well as the swine epidemic diarrhea virus and the transmissible gastroenteritis coronavirus.

Betacoronavirus genus.

Also known as Group 2 coronavirus. The most important are OC43 and HKU1 (type A); SARS-CoV and SARS-CoV-2 (type B) and MERS-CoV (type C).

15. Animal-borne coronaviruses

Coronaviruses of the Orthocoronavirinae subfamily are zoonotic pathogens, that is, they are closely linked to wild or farm animals. Of these, they pass to the human being through consumption of their meat or contact with their body fluids.

An example of animal-borne coronaviruses is SARS-CoV, which causes Severe Acute Respiratory Syndrome (SARS), a disease that can end in severe respiratory failure.

The first SARS-CoV case was reported in 2002 in Guangdong province, China. From there it spread to more than 30 countries with a total of 8,000 infected and 774 deaths.

Studies indicated that the primary source of SARS-CoV was civet cats, likely infected with bat bites. These cats were hunted for sale in live animal markets in China. The virus passed from cats to humans through consumption of their meat.

Another animal-borne coronavirus is MERS-CoV, which causes Middle East Respiratory Syndrome (MERS). In 2012, the first case of MERS was reported in Saudi Arabia, but it is considered that it possibly arose for the first time in Jordan earlier that year.

By 2019, he had already claimed 850 lives and sickened 2,500 people in various parts of the world, most of them from the Middle East or who had traveled to that part of the world.

The original reservoir for the MERS-CoV coronavirus is considered to have been camels, widely used in this part of the world as pack animals and sources of meat and milk.

For its part, the new SARS-CoV-2 coronavirus, which causes the new severe acute respiratory syndrome COVID-19, originates from horseshoe bats, a very abundant species in China and which is hunted for sale in markets in that country. .

In fact, the first cases of COVID-19 occurred in people who had visited or purchased products at the Wuhan City Seafood Wholesale Market, where live animals, including horseshoe bats, are sold.

16. Resistance in different environments

SARS-CoV-2 has shown a great ability to survive outside the body of the human or animal host. It can remain active for 4 days on glass surfaces, as well as five days on paper or cardboard objects. For leather and rubber objects, such as winter gloves and those worn by medical personnel, it can survive up to 8 hours.

Various studies have shown that it can be active for up to 6 hours on natural or synthetic fabrics, and up to 8 hours on aluminum surfaces. In addition, it can withstand temperatures of up to 38 degrees Celsius, facilitating its spread in hot climates to a much higher level than other known coronaviruses.

17. Differences between COVID-19 and previous coronaviruses

Although COVID-19 causes symptoms similar to SARS-CoV and MERS-CoV, the symptoms it causes and the way it spreads are slightly different from the latter two.

COVID-19 is transmitted primarily from person to person through body fluids, such as saliva, even at distances of 3 meters. In this it resembles MERS-CoV and SARS-CoV, but COVID-19 has greater resistance to the environment, including high temperature. However, its high survival capacity and contagion power is offset by a lower mortality rate.

While the number of infected by COVID-19 worldwide reached 850,583 people at the end of March 2020, the number of deaths only reached 41,654, which is equivalent to a mortality rate of 4.89% This is much less than the mortality rate of 35% of the MERS-CoV and 10% of the SARS-CoV outbreak.

18. Virulence of COVID-19

SARS-CoV-2 has a greater contagion capacity than any other coronavirus, as evidenced by the fact that just 3 months after the first confirmed case, more than 850,000 people had been infected in 190 countries and territories on the planet. In addition, its incubation period is 14 days, which increases the possibility that a patient will infect others before showing symptoms.

But in compensation, COVID-19 has a much lower mortality rate than MERS-CoV, SARS-CoV and Influenza. A study published in late March in The Lancet: Infectious Diseases, by British researchers who analyzed data from 70,117 cases diagnosed in China, indicated that the COVID-19 death rate is just 0.66% . This figure takes into account that many infections and deaths are not clinically confirmed. If only confirmed clinical cases are taken into account, the COVID-19 mortality rate rises to just 1.38%.

For its part, the China Center for Disease Control and Prevention revealed that studies done in Wuhan indicated that only 9.1% of COVID-19 patients showed severe to severe symptoms, while 80.9% had mild symptoms. or even remained asymptomatic.

The decisive factor in the mortality rate is the age of the patient, since the majority of deaths correspond to adults over 60 years of age with previous conditions such as diabetes, hypertension or immunosuppressive diseases.

Among deceased older adults, 8% are in the range of 60-80 years of age, but from the age of 80 these constitute 15% of registered deaths worldwide.

Some diseases also increase the death rate of COVID-19. Patients affected by cardiovascular problems have had a death rate of 10.5%. Among diabetics, deaths from COVID-19 represent 7.3% of cases.

Likewise, among the group of patients with previous chronic respiratory problems, the mortality rate from COVID-19 has remained at 6.3%.

19. Immunity to COVID-19

To date, there are no known cases of people cured of COVID-19 who have developed immunity to this disease. What is known is that some patients in China, Germany, Japan, and Italy who had recovered became ill again after becoming infected with new strains of SARS-CoV-2.

The first case of COVID-19 reinfection was reported in Japan, in a 70-year-old man who had been diagnosed with COVID-19 on February 14, 2020. After being hospitalized in Tokyo, the man recovered and was discharged. . But after a few days he felt sick again and was hospitalized again. Doctors found that SARS-CoV-2 was present again in his body. This case led to a harsh belief by scientists and researchers that no one could get COVID-19 twice in a row.

In late March 2020, the German government announced that it will study 100,000 healthy people who did not get sick despite being exposed to COVID-19 patients. The objective is to determine if they have any natural immunity that could be used to develop a COVID-19 vaccine or preventive medicine.

China, the United States, Germany and Russia are working on the development of vaccines against SARS-CoV-2, but it is estimated that none will be ready and definitively approved for mass application to the population before April 2021.

Meanwhile, drug therapies are applied for malaria and other diseases, which have given positive results in the relief of symptoms in the most serious patients.

Part III. Risk and transmission between humans

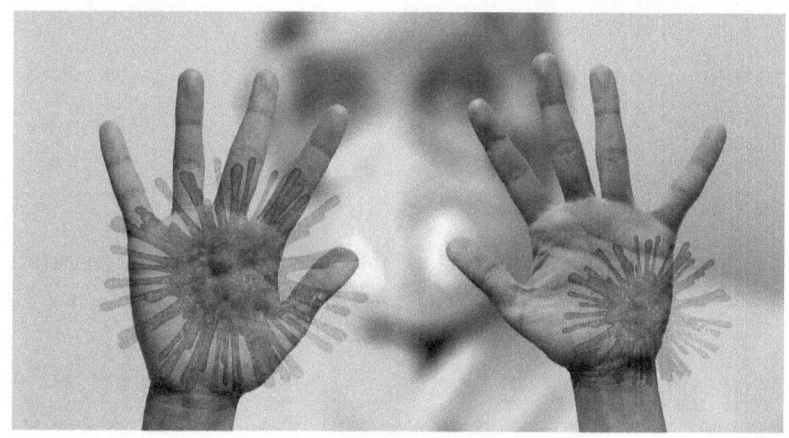

The COVID-19 outbreak is similar to the 2020 Severe Acute Respiratory Syndrome (SARS) and 2012 Middle East Respiratory Syndrome (MERS) outbreaks.

SARS and MERS appeared by zoonotic transmission related to bats, which infected civet cats (SARS) in Guangdong, China, as well as camels in Saudi Arabia (MERS).

In the case of COVID-19, it is related to the consumption of meat of horseshoe bats in the Hubei region, China.

20. Epidemiological characteristics

Several studies carried out in China and Europe during the months of February and March 2020 yielded interesting data on the epidemiological characteristics of this COVID-19 outbreak.

The incubation period has been determined to be 3 to 7 days and patient recovery can take 14 days in mild cases and 3 to 6 weeks in severe and critical cases. Very young patients tend to be relatively resistant to infection, with just 1% of those infected aged 10 to 19 years and 0.9% infected at ages younger than 10 years.

On the contrary, people with ages between 30 to 79 years constitute the bulk of positive cases, with 87% of all infected.

For their part, people between 20 and 29 years old have an infection rate of 8%, while in those over 80 years it increases to 18%.

Furthermore, it was determined that 1% of infected patients did not show any symptoms during the entire type they convalesced.

Another characteristic of COVID-19 is that despite being highly contagious, 81% of those infected only present mild symptoms, such as dry cough, fever and general tiredness, but they do not develop pneumonia or in any case only mild pneumonia.

On the other hand, only 14% of those infected present a serious clinical picture, with symptoms of dyspnea, respiratory rate greater than or equal to 30 inspirations per minute and blood oxygen saturation equal to or less than 93%.

They may also present partial pressure of arterial oxygen to fraction of inspired oxygen less than 300 or pulmonary infiltrates greater than 50%, all in a period of just 24 to 48 hours from the appearance of the first symptoms.

Likewise, COVID-19 patients who reach a critical state barely represent 5% of those infected.

These patients show symptoms of respiratory failure, septic shock and / or malfunction or total failure in multiple organs.

As for the mortality rate, it is highly influenced by the age of the patient. The COVID-19 pandemic has shown a fatality of 2.3% in China and 1.9% in the rest of the world, but this figure increases to 14.8% in the case of patients with age equal to or greater than 80 years. In the case of patients between the ages of 70 to 79 years, the mortality rate drops to 8.0%. It is also noteworthy that the probability of death among critically ill patients is 49.0%.

Additionally, the fatality rate increases considerably when the patient suffers from a pre-existing comorbid condition, regardless of age. In this regard, among those who died from COVID-19, it was found that 10.5% suffered from cardiovascular diseases, 7.3% were diabetic and 6.3% suffered from chronic lung diseases. For their part, hypertensive patients represented 6% of all fatal cases and oncological patients 5.6%.

21. Most common transmission routes

The World Health Organization (WHO) has reported that the most frequent transmission of COVID-19 between people is through droplets from the nose or mouth, which are expelled when breathing, speaking, coughing or sneezing.

The nasal droplets can be deposited on people or objects within a radius of 1 meter around the infected patient. For glass surfaces, the SARS-CoV-2 can be active for up to 4 days and up to 8 hours on metal, fabric, latex or leather surfaces.

According to studies carried out on infected patients, the most likely form of entry of COVID-19 into the human body is through the eyes, nose and mouth.

Infection through the eyes occurs both by contamination of the ocular conjunctiva with droplets expelled by an infected person, and by touching the hands after contact with a contaminated surface.

22. Transmission by air drops

On March 27, 2020, the WHO published a study that reiterates that the main form of transmission of COVID-19 from a sick person to a healthy person is by droplets expelled through the nose and mouth and by contact with contaminated surfaces.

When breathing or coughing, these droplets can move 1 meter away from the patient, reaching the mucosa of the nose and mouth, as well as the conjunctiva of the eyes of anyone nearby. They can also fall on objects and surfaces near the infected person, where COVID-19 can remain active from 6 hours to the following 4 days.

23. Transmission by direct contact

Studies conducted until the end of March 2020 have found no evidence that COVID-19 is transmitted by direct skin contact from an infected to a healthy patient. Furthermore, there appears to be a very low risk that contact with the feces of an infected person favors contagion, even though the SARS-CoV-2 coronavirus may be present in them. The WHO has indicated that there are still no known cases of fecal-oral transmission of COVID-19.

Therefore, transmission by droplets emanating from the nose and mouth and contact with contaminated objects and surfaces remains the main officially confirmed form of contagion. For this reason, the WHO insists on the need for the population to wash their hands frequently and avoid touching their eyes and nose.

24. Risks for closer contacts

The risk of COVID-19 coronavirus infection is directly related to the level of exposure. Close contacts of infected people face the highest risk of exposure through sharing bedding, towels, plates and cutlery, furniture and other everyday objects. Added to this is exposure to nasal droplet emissions from coughing, breathing, or sneezing. This especially includes family, couples, and coworkers.

Medical personnel caring for patients showing symptoms of COVID-19 also face a high risk of transmission, making it mandatory to wear appropriately certified protective suits, masks and gloves for high-risk infections.

The fact that a percentage of those infected do not have symptoms makes it more difficult to take measures in time to prevent the spread of their closest beings.

Furthermore, studies to date have not clarified when a person infected with COVID-19 becomes the focus of infection for others.

For this reason, the WHO recommends that relatives of anyone showing symptoms of SARS-CoV-2 be placed under immediate observation, even before the results of their analyzes are received.

For those who were discharged and show symptoms again, they need to be isolated immediately before they can become contagious again.

25. Medical observation of contacts for 14 days

Persons close to confirmed COVID-19 patients should be kept under medical observation for 14 days, the maximum time it takes for symptoms to manifest. However, the absence of symptoms does not exempt the need for laboratory tests, since many sick people may be asymptomatic.

The medical observation should preferably be carried out in a quarantine situation, either in the patient's home or in a properly prepared medical center to receive this type of patient.

26. Cutting the transmission chain

Social isolation is decisive in cutting the transmission chain of COVID-19, since it allows healthy individuals to be kept away from emissions of respiratory secretions from infected patients.

Disinfection of surfaces and objects close to COVID-19 patients is also important.

Following the example of the Chinese authorities, the WHO recommends disinfecting public spaces, streets and avenues, as well as furniture and objects for daily use using disinfectants based on chlorine, 75% alcohol and other lipid solvents.

Possible contaminated objects can also be disinfected by irradiating them with ultraviolet light and heat greater than 56°C for at least 30 minutes. Furthermore, it is important to comply with individual and collective hygiene measures to reduce the possibility of contagion.

The first is to wash your hands several times a day with soap and water or apply an alcohol-based gel. A distance of at least 1 meter should be maintained between person and person, especially if the other person frequently coughs or sneezes. You should also avoid touching your eyes, nose, and mouth, particularly after touching objects or surfaces on the street.

When sneezing or coughing, the mouth and nose should be covered with the inside of the elbow and not with the hands. Ideally, use a disposable tissue that should be removed immediately. If you have any symptoms of fever, cough and shortness of breath it is best to stay home and inform the emergency numbers if these symptoms worsen. The indications and updated information offered by the local or national health authorities must be followed, both on the progress of COVID-19 and on what must be done to protect against it.

27. Risk groups more susceptible to contagion

Health personnel are the group most at risk of becoming infected with COVID-19, given that it occupies the first level of care for suspected cases.

In addition, they work in spaces where the accumulation of infected patients makes it more likely that there will be contaminated surfaces and objects. For example, in March 2020, the Spanish government recorded 5,600 infected doctors and health workers from COVID-19.

Second are people who work in companies that serve large numbers of the public, such as employees of stores, supermarkets, cinemas and collective recreation sites.

For their part, researchers from the Evidence-Based Medicine Center and the Zhongnan Hospital of Wuhan University found that among the patients who died from COVID-19, 42% had type A blood.

In turn, they found that only 25% of the deceased had type O blood, which suggests a relationship between blood type and vulnerability to contagion of the person.

Age also influences vulnerability to contagion. Infants and children under the age of 10 appear to be highly resistant to contagion, while adults over the age of 60 are highly vulnerable.

However, this disease can attack anyone and given the conditions of each person, it can be fatal.

Part IV Cases, clinic and possible complications

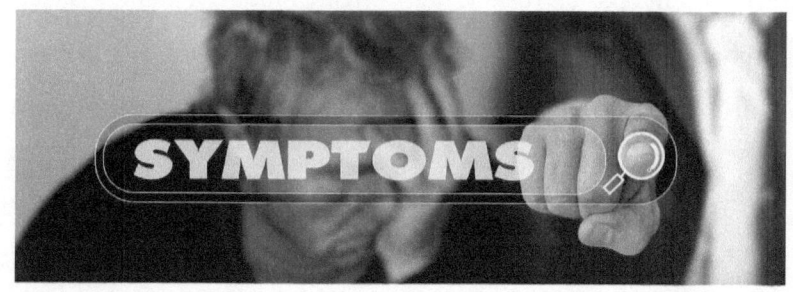

28. Subclinical cases

Subclinical cases of COVID-19 refer to patients who have been infected with the SARS-CoV-2 coronavirus but still show no symptoms. This group is the object of special attention by the researchers, since it is still unknown at what moment from the initial contagion, an asymptomatic infected patient can become contagious.

The SARS-CoV-2 virus has an average incubation period of 5 days, but less than 2.5% of people will show any symptoms within the first 60 hours from the time of exposure.

In the vast majority of cases, COVID-19 symptoms appear 12 to 14 days after the initial infection, and in some cases there will never be symptoms, even if the person has a high viral load in the blood. There is also a chance that symptoms will appear after the 2-week quarantine period that applies to most suspected cases.

This represents a great challenge for those responsible for controlling the COVID-19 pandemic, as indicated by a study published in the Annals of Internal Medicine.

According to the trial, 101 out of 10,000 cases will only show symptoms after exiting 14-day active surveillance.

29. Suspicious cases

As the initial outbreak of COVID-19 intensified in the city of Wuhan, China, in January 2020, the Zhongnan Hospital of that city recommended that any individual who visited that city after December 15 be classified as a "suspicious case" However, in a few weeks the outbreak spread throughout China and from there to the rest of the world.

Therefore, anyone who has traveled to an area where COVID-19 cases have been reported or who has had direct contact with someone from it came to be considered a "suspected case".

Subsequently, given the increase in community infections in a large number of countries, this qualification began to be applied to anyone who presented one or more of the initial symptoms of COVID-19, such as fever, physical fatigue, dry cough and sore throat.

30. Confirmed cases

On April 3, 2020, just a month and a half after declaring the COVID-19 pandemic, the WHO reported that the number of people infected by this virus in the world was 971,591 people.

In addition, the number of deaths that day reached 75,853 and the number of recovered patients rose to 50,311. These figures corresponded to the information provided by the health governing bodies of the different nations, but it was not necessarily the actual number of people infected.

The main problem in obtaining reliable figures for infections, deaths and recoveries is that many countries do not have COVID-19 early detection systems that can be applied to 100% of the population.

In addition, in each country, different criteria are applied to measure death rates from diseases. For example, the Chinese government was accused at the time of concealing the actual number of infected and deceased in the initial outbreak in Wuhan City.

In Germany and the Nordic countries, for example, many initial deaths from COVID-19 were recorded as being caused by other underlying conditions such as coronary heart disease, acute respiratory failure, pneumonia, sepsis, and kidney failure. This was particularly evident in the case of older adults.

Another case was that of Ecuador, where a notable increase in deaths of older adults was reported in the Guayas region. These died in their homes after presenting obvious respiratory symptoms and without receiving help from health entities or being subsequently examined to verify if the cause of death was SARS-CoV-2.

Although Ecuador officially reported at that time a total of 120 victims of COVID-19, the estimates of the Ecuadorian medical unions is that the real number was close to 450 deaths.

This led the WHO to request governments to stricter follow-up of suspected cases and the application of policies that guarantee the care of the population, especially in the most vulnerable social sectors.

31. Most common symptoms of the disease

COVID-19 disease has relatively mild symptoms compared to Influenza, SARS, and MERS. In many cases, even no symptoms are manifested.

Infected people manifest the first symptoms within 2 to 5 days after exposure and in some cases 14 days or more.

According to statistics collected in China during the month of February 2020 based on the analysis of 55,924 confirmed cases of COVID-19, the most common symptoms and the percentage with which they manifest are:

- Recurrent fever equal to or greater than 38°C (87.9% of cases)
- Dry cough (67.7%)
- Physical tiredness or fatigue (38.1%)
- For its part, in moderate to severe cases symptoms such as:
- Dyspnea or shortness of breath (18.6%)
- Muscle and joint pain (14.8%)
- Sore throat (13.9%)
- Headache (13.6%)
- Chills (11.4%)

In some cases vomiting (5%) and diarrhea (3.7%) occur even before the above symptoms appear.

A frequently reported symptom, even in asymptomatic patients, is the sudden loss of the senses of taste and smell.

32. Clinical signs to look for

When evaluating a person suspected of being infected with COVID-19, the presence of clinical signs such as recurrent or persistent fever equal to or greater than 38°C, permanent fatigue, low white blood cell count and low level of T cells (lymphopenia) should be sought.

It is also important to assess the presence of pneumonia or some form of dyspnea caused by the accumulation of sputum in the lungs.

33. Important laboratory tests

In addition to the early identification of symptoms in people suspected of having COVID-19, there are several tests recommended by the WHO and research centers in China and Europe.

One of these is the blood test to determine if the levels of leukocytes and T cells in the blood have decreased, since it has been found that unlike other infections, COVID-19 causes a loss of the response capacity of the immune system.

Radiological examinations of the patient's lungs are also important to determine the presence of pneumonia and / or obstruction of the bronchi due to excessive accumulation of sputum.

The WHO has issued some protocols for the rapid diagnosis of COVID-19. One of them, applied in Japan, is the Quantitative Polymerase Chain Reaction and Reaction in Real Time Test (RT-PCR). This test is performed on samples taken from the patient's upper respiratory tract or blood and can give a result in a few hours.

Another rapid test to detect COVID-19 is based on the detection of IgG and IgM antibodies against SARS-CoV-2 present in samples of blood, blood plasma or serum.

This method was developed in China and can give results in just 15 minutes.

On March 14, 2020, the President of the United States, Donald Trump, announced that the Roche company had developed a new analysis system based on the qualitative detection of SARS-CoV-2 in samples taken from the nasopharyngeal and oropharyngeal mucosa of suspected patients. . This test, as reported, can give a definitive result in just 3 ½ hours.

34. X-rays and chest tomography

Chest radiographs and tomographies are determining tools for the early diagnosis of COVID-19 in patients affected by pneumonia and other symptoms suspected of being infected with SARS-CoV-2.

On March 12, 2020, the Radiological Society of North America released the first images from an X-ray study of the lungs of a COVID-19 fatality.

The images showed the victim's lungs, a 44-year-old man, 70 percent full of mucous material.

The presence of large white spots called "ground glass opacities" stood out, covering the lower area of both lungs. These opacities resemble those seen in SARS-CoV and

MERS-CoV patients who developed severe symptoms of pneumonia.

On the other hand, the CT scans made of other patients who died from COVID-19 showed that this disease causes a partial filling of the alveoli and bronchi with a large amount of phlegm, causing severe respiratory failure.

Econosography has also been very valuable in the pulmonary evaluation of patients in health centers where there are not enough computed tomography or X-ray equipment.

Currently, and because there are already rapid tests to confirm the presence of COVID-19, these radiological and ultrasound techniques are mainly used in the clinical evaluation of damage suffered by patients' lungs.

35. Mild complications

COVID-19 disease is associated with serious infections in the lungs, which can affect any patient, regardless of age or previous physical conditions.

However, more than 80% of patients only experience mild or moderate symptoms.

The most common complications are related to impaired lung function due to mild pneumonia.

In addition, air flow is reduced due to the presence of phlegm in the bronchi and bronchioles, which reduces the level of oxygenation of the blood.

In mild cases, the complications of COVID-19 are:

- Difficulty breathing and / or shortness of breath
- Chest pain and constant feeling of pressure in the chest
- Mental confusion and / or difficulties waking up from sleep
- Appearance of a bluish tone on nails, lips and face

In general terms, in most cases the complications of COVID-19 are the same as the flu or influenza and people recovered from the infection do not have major sequelae.

36. Serious complications

For people over 60, COVID-19 can cause serious complications that can lead to death.

This also occurs with patients of any age who have previous underlying conditions such as high blood pressure, diabetes, chronic kidney disease, cancer and chronic respiratory disease, among others.

People undergoing cancer treatment and those with Acquired Immune Deficiency Syndrome (AIDS) are especially susceptible to developing serious complications because their immune systems are weakened.

As the WHO has reported, 15% of people infected with COVID-19 will present a severe condition, while 5% will develop critical complications that will force them to be put on intensive therapy. Of this group, just over 50% can die from the systemic damage caused by this disease.

Some of the serious complications of COVID-19 patients are:

Bilateral pulmonary pneumonia of different degrees, with the presence of ground glass opacity on X-ray images and tomography.

Acute Respiratory Failure Syndrome due to obstruction of the airways due to the production of abundant thick phlegm and inflammation of the pleural membrane.

Insufficiency or failure in the function of one or more organs, such as kidneys, liver, brain and heart.

Another possible serious complication of COVID-19 is the appearance of a picture of bacterial pneumonia, promoted by the drop in the body's defenses due to the action of the SARS-CoV-2 coronavirus on the immune system.

In very severe cases, septic shock may occur due to failure of the function of major organs combined with secondary infections in the lungs and intestines. This septic shock can present simultaneously to the Acute Respiratory Failure Syndrome, which places the patient in a situation of extreme danger.

37. Other complications

Some rare complications of COVID-19 are the appearance of hemoptysis, or the presence of blood in the pulmonary sputum. This complication has only been registered in 0.9% of patients, but for the most part the blood comes from the pharyngeal area, severely irritated by the cough.

Other minor complications are diarrhea, which occurs in 3.7% of those infected, as well as vomiting, which affects 5% of patients. These complications, although not fatal, can affect the patient's mood and cause moderate to severe dehydration and malnutrition if not treated in time.

In 0.8% of cases, a strong picture of eye irritation can also occur, especially in the early stages of the disease. This symptom usually accompanies nasal congestion and sore throat that affect many patients.

Part V. Community-acquired pneumonia

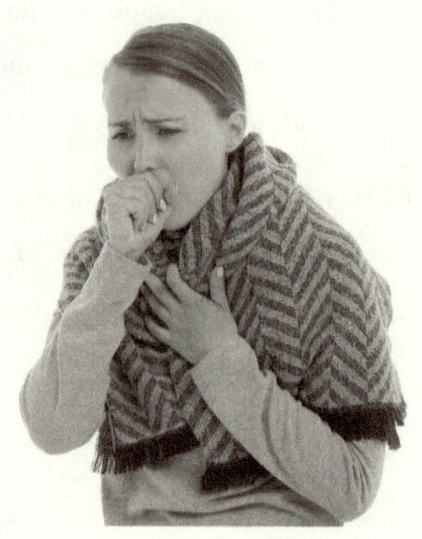

Pneumonia can be caused by various types of germs, but the most common are viruses, fungi, and bacteria in the air.

Clinically, pneumonia is classified based on the type of pathogen that causes it.

38. Concepts

Pneumonia is a picture of the respiratory system characterized by the presence of inflammation of the air sacs of one or both lungs, caused by an infection or the action of an external agent. These air sacs, or alveoli, can be filled with liquid or purulent material as a result of the body's inflammatory response and the activation of the cells responsible for fighting the pathogen.

Pneumonia is usually accompanied by symptoms such as pain and shortness of breath, fever, chills, and cough accompanied by abundant phlegm. Pneumonia is classified by cause, which can be a bacterial agent, a virus, fungi, or the entry of a foreign substance or body into the lungs.

Although it is common for hospital patients to develop pneumonia as a consequence of their clinical symptoms, the majority of reported cases in the world correspond to community-acquired pneumonia.

These by definition are those respiratory infections that are acquired in the environment where the patient lives and works.

39. Difference with nosocomial pneumonia

It is important to differentiate community-acquired pneumonia from nosocomial pneumonia. The contagion that causes nosocomial pneumonia (NN) occurs during the stay in a greeting center or hospital and manifests between 48 to 72 hours after the patient is discharged.

The main danger of nosocomial pneumonia is that it is caused by the action of bacterial strains that have developed resistance to most antibiotics by passing from one sick individual to another in a cycle repeated numerous times.

Those people who are affected by their immune system due to illness, injury or medications and who receive assisted breathing for long periods of time are more likely to get nosocomial pneumonia. This condition is also valid for patients undergoing dialysis, as well as healthcare personnel who spend long hours in these health centers.

For its part, community-acquired pneumonia is usually due to the action of bacteria or viruses present in the environment, which have not always developed resistance to modern antibiotics. The appearance of the outbreak is usually related to the previous spread of influenza or influenza between healthy and sick people who share the same environment.

40. Diagnostic criteria

The diagnosis of pneumonia is mainly based on the presence of symptoms such as high fever, cough and chest pain or pleuritic pain.

X-ray images will show large white spots on the lobes of one or both lungs, as well as possible signs of pleural effusion. A picture of pneumonia can also be determined by the blood oxygen and leukocyte values.

In cases where bacterial pneumonia is suspected, sputum or mucus cultures can be done to identify the pathogen and determine the antibiotic to use. Today there are urine tests to detect pneumococcal and legionella antigen.

In severe cases, a lung puncture can be performed to free fluid accumulated in the pleural wall and samples can be taken, as well as a bronchoscopy to sample mucus from the lower respiratory tract.

41. Causal pathogenic bacteria

In the United States, the most common cause of community-acquired pneumonia is infection with the Streptococcus pneumoniae bacteria.

This type of infection usually occurs in patients who have just had a serious cold or flu, as their immune system is temporarily weakened. However, it can also occur without a previous respiratory condition having occurred.

Bacterial pneumonia can affect one or both lungs. It can also occur only in one lobe of the lung or in the entire organ.

HIV / AIDS patients often contract pneumonia from the action of the Pneumocystis bacteria.

A second type of bacterial pneumonia is caused by Mycoplasma pneumoniae. This medical condition is often called wandering pneumonia, since its symptoms are milder than those caused by Streptococcus pneumoniae infection.

Because of this, many patients do not require rest or hospital care and can recover within a few days. Although they are not bacteria, fungi are one of the most frequent causes of pathogenic origin of pneumonia.

These fungi are present in garden and field soils, or in areas where large amounts of bird feces are deposited. They are more abundant in hot and humid climate regions. The more fungus a person inhales in these environments, the greater the probability of developing pneumonia.

42. Risk factors and prevention

Pneumonia can attack any individual, regardless of age or sex. However, children under 2 years of age and adults over 65 are the most likely social groups to suffer from this condition. In addition to age, there are risk factors that can increase the possibility of pneumonia.

These include the following:

- Having chronic obstructive pulmonary disease (COPD) or asthma.
- Suffering from heart disease.

- Being hospitalized for a long time in an intensive care unit, particularly if you are receiving ventilator-assisted breathing.
- Being a chronic smoker or being exposed to cigarette smoke for many hours a day (passive smoker).
- Having an autoimmune disease or that weakens the immune system.

People affected by cystic fibrosis can develop pneumonia frequently due to the continuous accumulation of fluid in their lungs, which, among other things, favors the growth of bacteria that enter the upper airways.

People affected by HIV / AIDS, as well as lung, kidney or liver transplant patients, who have weak immune systems due to illness and consumption of anti-rejection medications, respectively, are also particularly vulnerable to pneumonia.

Cancer patients undergoing radiotherapy and chemotherapy are also considered high risk for pneumonia, as well as those suffering from inflammatory diseases that require the use of steroids for a long period of time.

The habit of smoking is a factor that favors the appearance of recursive pneumonia, since the chemicals present in the cigarette damage the pulmonary epithelium, where the beards or cilia that sweep the dust particles and dead cells are located outside the lungs.

The best prevention that can be done against pneumonia is the same as that applied for any other disease transmitted by bacteria or viruses. This includes washing your hands several times a day with soap and water or an alcohol-based solution.

This should be done especially if you have contact with surfaces touched by large numbers of people, such as restaurant tables, bars, doors, etc.

People who show symptoms of a cold or severe cough should also avoid waving handshake. In this case, it is advisable to maintain a minimum distance of one meter with the person who shows respiratory symptoms, however slight they may be.

43. Viral pneumonia

Some of the viruses responsible for influenza can cause pneumonia, especially in children younger than 5 years and adults older than 65 years. This occurs because their organisms have less ability to fight the action of viruses, which increases the possibility that they affect the lungs.

Viral pneumonia can be caused by one of the following viruses:

- Influenza virus
- Parainfluenza virus
- Respiratory Syncytial Virus (RSV)
- Adenovirus
- Measles virus

Furthermore, the patients who most frequently develop viral pneumonia are:

- Premature babies
- Infants under the age of 10 with lung or heart problems
- People infected with HIV / AIDS
- Cancer patients undergoing chemotherapy, radiotherapy or medications that affect the immune system.

- People who have undergone an organ transplant and take anti-rejection medications.

Generally speaking, pneumonias caused by viruses have mild to moderate symptoms and only in certain cases lead to severe cases that endanger the patient's life.

44. Pneumonia due to COVID-19

Despite having a much higher contagion capacity than other diseases caused by coronavirus, COVID-19 disease usually presents mild symptoms. In most cases, those infected only have a dry cough, sore throat, shortness of breath and a fever of 38°C.

Only in moderate or severe cases develops a picture of pneumonia. In these cases, the chances of death are greatly increased if the patient is elderly or suffers from another underlying disease.

COVID-19 pneumonia is characterized by an excessive accumulation of fluid and phlegm in the lungs, which practically reduces its capacity to oxygenate the blood to less than 30%.

X-ray images and CT scans of COVID-19 patients with pneumonia pictures show large opaque areas called "ground glass opacity", indicating severe obstruction of alveoli, bronchioles, and bronchi.

45. Differences with other pneumonias

Pneumonia caused by COVID-19 disease represents a serious risk to the life of the patient if it is not treated in time. More than 50% of the deaths recorded in the Chinese city of Wuhan during the first 60 days of the COVID-19 outbreak corresponded to older adults who developed severe symptoms of pneumonia.

For their part, people who did not suffer from pneumonia recovered in about two weeks in almost 80% of cases and no major sequelae were seen. This contrasts with other coronavirus-induced pneumonias such as the 2012 MERS-CoV and the 2002 SARS-CoV, where there was a lower infection rate but much higher mortality.

In both outbreaks, 75% of those infected developed viral pneumonia and the people recovered suffered sequels that included the permanent loss of up to 30% of their respiratory capacity due to damage to their lung tissues.

46. Severe acute respiratory syndrome

Severe acute respiratory syndrome (SARS) is a disease of the respiratory system caused by the SARS-CoV-2 coronavirus, as well as other infectious or non-infectious diseases.

Being the final complication of the disease, COVID-19 is contagious and can be fatal. It was recently described in China in 2002 and spread through various countries through infected travelers, in the outbreak of the SARS-CoV-1 epidemic.

This disease has flu-like symptoms, including dry cough, shortness of breath, fever of 38°C and chills, muscle aches, headache, and sometimes vomiting and diarrhea.

Thanks to the international effort, the outbreak could be contained and since 2004 there have been no new cases of SARS by SARS-Cov-1 in the world.

47. Respiratory sepsis and septic shock

Patients affected by pneumonia, as in the case of COVID-19, SARS and MERS, can develop a severe infectious process that in turn causes an extreme defensive reaction of the organism.

The production of leukocytes and phlegm is increased to try to expel infectious agents from the lungs and these fill with fluid as an allergic response to the infection.

These conditions can favor the development of respiratory sepsis, due to the proliferation of opportunistic bacteria in the warm, moist environment of the lungs. In turn, the infection can pass into the patient's blood and affect organs such as the heart, liver, intestine, and kidneys.

The organism enters a state of septic shock due to the accumulation of toxins produced by bacteria and viruses, as well as the failure of the kidneys and liver, responsible for filtering the blood.

48. Extra respiratory complications

People affected by pneumonia can develop complications that affect the function of organs other than the lungs.

The most common in severe pneumonia is bacteremia, which occurs when bacteria that infect the lungs pass into the bloodstream and spread to other organs.

Bacteremia can cause a picture of organ failure and sepsis that can be fatal in children and older adults.

49. Multiple organ failure

As mentioned above, pneumonia at its most severe stage can lead to bacteremia, which is the spread of the lung infection into the blood and from there to organs such as the liver, heart, brain, kidneys, and intestine.

An uncontrolled infection can cause failure of one or more of these organs, which in turn increases the accumulation of toxins and metabolic waste in the body. Kidney failure is one of the first consequences of severe pneumonia, followed by liver failure.

In addition, many antibiotics used in the fight against bacterial pneumonia can have harmful effects on the liver and kidneys and contribute to its failure in the short and medium term.

50. Medical discharge for pneumonia

Patients with pneumonia are discharged when the inflammatory process in the lungs ceases and clinical examinations indicate that the infection has subsided after treatment with antibiotics and rest.

However, this does not mean that the patient will be completely healthy, since there are several symptoms and sequelae that require more time to disappear.

The cough associated with pneumonia usually takes 1 to 2 weeks to fully improve. Appetite and sleep can be affected for up to 1 week after the pneumonia symptoms have subsided.

In addition to this, muscle pain and a feeling of physical tiredness can last up to a month from the discharge of the pneumonia patient.

In most cases, doctors will give patients a 30-day rest to promote their full recovery from such a condition.

Part VI. High risk of mortality

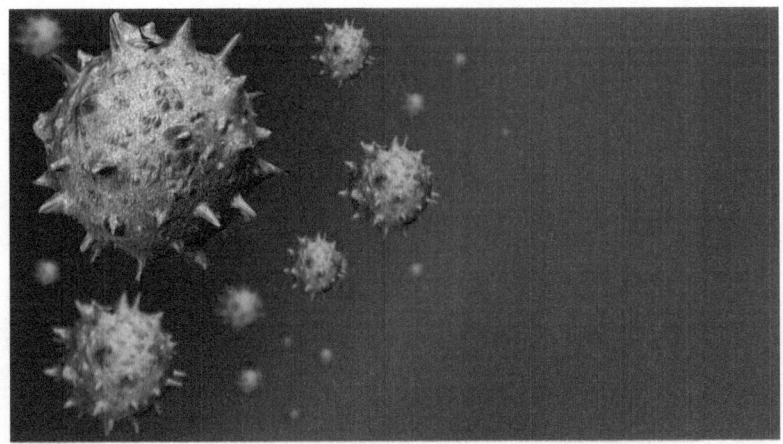

51. Cardiovascular diseases

A study published by the American College of Cardiology noted that cardiovascular disease patients who contract COVID-19 have a death rate of 10.5%. This corresponds to observations made in previous outbreaks of coronavirus diseases, where it was found that the most severe patients also tended to have cardiovascular injuries or problems.

In addition, patients without previous heart problems developed this type of ailment when their symptoms reached a critical level, in which they needed intensive care.

Among the complications that can affect severe patients with COVID-19 are arrhythmias, acute coronary syndromes and the appearance or exacerbation of heart failure.

COVID-19 causes a process of vasculitis, or inflammation of the blood vessels, as well as an inflammation of the middle layer of the heart muscle, called myocarditis.

Data obtained from clinical cases of COVID-19 in Wuhan, China, as well as in the United States, indicate that people over 65 years of age with hypertension or coronary heart disease are more likely to contract SARS-CoV-2 serious disease and develop symptoms.

Global studies indicate a relationship between Troponin T (TnT) levels and the mortality rate of cardiac patients infected with COVID-19. The higher the TnT level, the greater the probability of developing a critical picture and even dying from COVID-19.

52. Elderly people

The mortality rate of COVID-19 is relatively low compared to other previous coronavirus diseases such as SARS (2002) and MERS (2012).

Globally, until March 2020, only 0.66 percent of those infected between the ages of 20 and 40 died from complications derived from COVID-19. However, in China, it had already been detected that this percentage increased dramatically in the range of 70 to 78 years of age, where mortality rose to 8%.

In turn, among patients older than 80 years, the mortality rate rose to 14.8%.

Furthermore, it was found that half of the fatal cases corresponded to adults over 60 years, many of whom suffered from other previous conditions such as diabetes, hypertension, cancer or kidney or liver deficiencies.

Studies conducted in the framework of the advance of the pandemic in Europe and the United States confirmed that older adults are more susceptible to developing severe symptoms or dying.

53. Smokers

Preliminary studies indicate that active and passive smokers are at greater risk of complications if they are infected with COVID-19 than other respiratory patients, such as asthmatics.

Specialists from around the world agree that tobacco produces a reaction in the lung tissue that favors the binding mechanism of the SARS-CoV-2 coronavirus with the cells of the lungs and therefore increases the speed of contagion.

Five trials conducted by Chinese universities during January and February 2020 found that, as with the flu or influenza, smokers are twice as likely to get COVID-19 than a nonsmoker of the same age.

One reason is that smoking causes permanent damage to the lung epithelium, responsible for protecting the lungs from infection, as well as expelling dust, bacteria, and dead cells.

In addition, the SARS-CoV-2 coronavirus has been found to survive up to 3 hours on surfaces such as copper and cardboard, as well as suspended in microdroplets from aerosols and in tobacco smoke and new electronic cigarettes.

This implies that a COVID-19 infected smoker can infect anyone nearby who breathes in the expired smoke, which will carry the active virus.

Statistical analysis of thousands of COVID-19 sufferers in Wuhan and other Chinese cities indicated that smoking patients developed severe to severe symptoms more frequently than nonsmokers.

In addition, smokers were also the group that most required assisted breathing and intensive care in severe cases, with 16.9% of cases, against 7.6% who were ex-smokers and 5.2% who never consumed tobacco.

To this it is added that smokers represented 25.8% of the deceased against 11.8% in the case of non-smokers.

54. Alcoholism

Alcohol addiction has consequences on the immune system, which exposes the person to a higher rate of infections by viruses such as the new COVID-19.

Additionally, alcohol nullifies the effect of most antibiotics and antiviral drugs used in the treatment of pneumonia and secondary infections caused by COVID-19.

In some cases, alcohol increases the toxicity and side effects of certain medications, which can affect kidney and liver function.

To this is added that a part of the alcohol that enters the body is expelled through respiration, irritating the lung tissue.

55. Bronchial asthma

Asthma is an inflammatory process of the respiratory system produced by an immune response of the body to both physical and emotional factors.

Bronchial asthma is considered a condition that considerably increases the risk of contracting COVID-19 and developing serious symptoms. In chronic asthmatics, inflammatory cells can cause acute damage to the lungs.

In those infected with COVID-19, the virus causes a dry cough and difficulty breathing because more phlegm or mucus is generated and fluid accumulates in the lungs.

This can pose a serious risk to asthmatic patients, who can develop an acute inflammatory process and require intensive care, assisted breathing or even die from total failure of the respiratory system.

56. Chronic lung disease

Patients affected by diseases of the respiratory system such as Chronic Obstructive Pulmonary Disease (COPD), Idiopathic Pulmonary Fibrosis (IPF) and asthma can present several symptoms very similar to those of COVID-19 disease.

These symptoms include dyspnea, dry cough, and general malaise. In many cases these patients do not seek medical attention when getting COVID-19 because they believe that their symptoms correspond to their previous lung conditions.

People with chronic lung disease face a serious risk if they get COVID-19, as this disease can cause moderate to severe pneumonia.

Additionally, COVID-19 causes severe diffuse injury throughout the lung, further reducing the blood oxygen level in people affected by underlying lung diseases.

Patients with severe pneumonia from COVID-19 who manage to recover may present permanent lung damage that reduces their respiratory capacity by up to 30%.

This is serious in a previously healthy and physically fit individual, but much more in the case of those who already suffered a decrease in their respiratory capacity due to other chronic lung diseases.

57. Diabetes mellitus

People over 60 years of age, as well as those with previous conditions such as asthma, diabetes mellitus, and heart problems, represent the group with the highest risk of complications and death from COVID-19.

When analyzing the data of more than 10,000 infected in the Chinese city of Wuhan, it was found that diabetics represented up to 20% of those infected who developed severe and severe symptoms.

In turn, among the most severe cases, diabetics reached a mortality rate of 7.3%. This is far higher than the death rate among the seriously infected without diabetes or other underlying diseases, which was just 0.9%.

One reason for this high mortality rate of diabetics infected with COVID-19 is that they have a greater tendency to develop viral infections because their immune system is compromised.

These people have white blood cells with a reduced phagocytosis capacity, which complicates their response to the presence of SARS-CoV-2 and lengthens the time necessary for recovery from an infection.

Added to this is that both SARS-CoV-2 and other viruses can thrive faster in individuals with high blood glucose levels.

Additionally, diabetes patients produce less amount of interferon, a molecule of great importance in the organic response to viruses, as well as CD8 or cytotoxic dysfunction.

58. Obesity

Obesity is not itself a fatal risk factor for a COVID-19 infection, but the diseases related to this condition are risks factors, such as diabetes, hypertension and respiratory problems.

Statistical studies by the U.S. Centers for Disease Control found that in the city of New Orleans the fatality rate from COVID-19 doubled that of New York State, despite having fewer confirmed cases.

This was because many of the patients in New Orleans were people who were overweight than 12 kilograms or morbidly obese and suffered from previous conditions such as hypertension, diabetes and asthma. Another reason that obese people with COVID-19 have a greater chance of dying if their condition worsens is that they have weaker immune systems than the average, overweight person.

In addition, a large percentage of obese people suffer from sleep apnea, a condition that affects their breathing during sleep and causes a drop in blood oxygen levels.

In addition, in many cases the transportation of an obese person complicated with COVID-19 is more difficult or even requires a great effort to get them out of their home and take them to a health center on time.

Another problem they face is the difficulty to perform tomography and X-ray plates, as well as to intubate them or get them a suitable bed for their weight and body size in case they require intensive care.

59. Hypothyroidism

Hypothyroidism is a condition in which the thyroid gland produces fewer hormones than normal. At least 5% of the world population is considered to suffer from hypothyroidism.

In the face of the COVID-19 pandemic, these types of patients have a mortality risk that varies depending on how the disease has manifested itself.

People with deficiency in their thyroid tend to develop overweight, a condition that in turn leads to hypertensive problems and blood circulation in the lower extremities. People with hypothyroidism not only gain weight without having increased food intake, but also often suffer from chronic fatigue or lack of energy.

The most frequent cause of hypothyroidism is the so-called Hashimoto's disease, in which the immune system attacks the thyroid. This causes permanent inflammation of the thyroid and a dysfunction in the production of hormones.

Other causes are radiation therapy treatments, side effects of some medications for liver or kidney ailments or for congenital causes.

In general, the mortality rate of these patients when taking COVID-19 is not directly related to the problem of their thyroid, but due to the deterioration in the general physical conditions of their organism derived from this.

60. Suprarrenal insufficiency

People suffering from adrenal insufficiency are prone to developing severe to severe conditions if they contract COVID-19, because their body is particularly vulnerable to infection or injury.

This is because your adrenal glands cannot produce the required amount of hormones like aldosterone and cortisol, which are involved in balancing blood pressure and blood glucose level.

Furthermore, this problem also alters the mechanism by which the body maintains the relationship between water and salt in the blood.

One of the consequences of this is that the body loses its ability to fight viral or bacterial infections.

In addition, the recovery from injuries or diseases in muscle, connective or bone tissues slows down.

In both cases of primary adrenal insufficiency (Addison's disease) or secondary adrenal insufficiency (due to hypopituitarism), treatments are usually based on glucocorticoid intake.

If the patient develops a dry cough and fever, as in severe to severe cases of COVID-19, the dose is usually doubled until symptoms subside. However, in some cases of severe

COVID-19 patients it has been noted that they are as vulnerable to bacterial and viral infections as diabetic patients, considered high risk.

In addition, glucocorticoids prescribed to control adrenal insufficiency can affect the body's immune response, so if the person contracts COVID-19, they would be vulnerable to pathogens that could aggravate their respiratory symptoms and cause organ failure.

61. Chronic kidney disease

The International Society of Nephrology (SIN) has reported that COVID-19 has not yet been shown to cause alterations in kidney function in patients with mild or moderate symptoms. However, in COVID-19 patients with severe symptoms and requiring hospitalization, a 25 to 50% loss of kidney function has been found.

Urine tests in these patients show signs of kidney damage, such as proteinuria and hematuria. Increased creatinine and urea nitrogen levels are also detected on your blood tests.

This confirms previous theories that indicate that the SARS-CoV-2 coronavirus can affect the kidneys because the cells of these, as well as of the lungs, have cells with receptors called ECA2, especially related to the protuberances or spikes of the outer layer of the coronavirus. This helps the virus infect these cells and multiply at a fast pace.

However, the SIN has indicated that less than 15% of COVID-19 patients develop a picture of acute kidney injury.

In any case, the SIN recommends monitoring the renal function of all those infected with COVID-19, whether or not they have previous chronic kidney disease, using the Glomerular Filtration Rate (GFR). The care of patients with chronic kidney disease who receive dialysis in health centers where they are infected with COVID-19.

These patients can develop nosocomial pneumonias and in themselves tend to have a decreased immune function that makes them prone to severe symptoms if they become infected with COVID-19.

62. HIV / AIDS

Carriers of the Human Immunodeficiency Virus (HIV) who are in good health have the same risk of becoming infected with COVID-19 as healthy people of the same age. If the HIV carrier is infected with COVID-19 but does not have other previous pathologies, it will show an evolution similar to that of any other person without HIV.

In the event that the patient has developed Acquired Immune Deficiency Syndrome (AIDS), caused by HIV, the risk of infection and complication increases substantially. It happens that the body loses the ability to defend itself against infections by fungi, bacteria and viruses.

The chances of surviving COVID-19 will depend on the patient's level of immunodeficiency, the type of treatment they are receiving, and their age.

It is noteworthy that antiviral drugs used in the treatment of HIV-AIDS have so far not been shown to have a protective effect against COVID-19.

There is also no evidence that chelopinavir, ritonavir, and other protease inhibitor drugs have a protective effect against SARS-CoV-2 entering the cells of the infected person.

In this regard, the European health authorities recommend that these patients take the prescribed dose of antivirals, whether or not they have COVID-19, and refrain from changing it outside the recommendation of the treating doctors.

Unfortunately, some 15 million people with HIV do not have access to antiviral drugs, according to the United Nations (UN).

63. Trasplanted

Patients who have received kidney, liver, heart and lung transplants are considered high risk for COVID-19.

As part of the post-operative process of a transplant, these people must take immunosuppressive medications, which reduce the responsiveness of the immune system. This is a way to prevent this system from attacking the transplanted organ, which you would consider as a foreign body.

This makes the patient more vulnerable to the action of SARS-CoV-2 and to any other bacteria or virus. In cases of organ transplant recipients who are infected with COVID-

19, the recommended treatment is to lower the dose of immunosuppressants as soon as symptoms of the disease appear, so that they have the opportunity to protect themselves from secondary infections.

64. Steroid use

Corticosteroid-based medications were used with mixed results in the treatment of patients with severe acute respiratory syndrome (SARS) in 2002 and Middle Eastern respiratory syndrome (MERS) in 2012.

Although steroids have been used in some European health centers in the treatment of COVID-19 pneumonia, the World Health Organization has discouraged their use where possible.

One of the reasons is that corticosteroids reduce the inflammatory process linked to infection in the COVID-19 patient's lungs.

This theoretically helps reduce the risk of acute lung injury and respiratory distress associated with moderate and severe cases of COVID-19 pneumonia.

However, corticosteroids also reduce the responsiveness of the immune system, which favors infections by bacteria or viruses, increasing the risk of septic shock or organ failure.

Furthermore, the benefit of anti-inflammatory steroid treatment in processes affecting the lungs as aggressively as COVID-19 is not yet clear. For this reason, the WHO recommends waiting for new studies that clarify the convenience or not of the use of steroids in the treatment of patients with this disease.

65. Immunosuppressed

Immunosuppressed patients are those whose immune system is weakened by a genetic condition, disease, or by the action of a drug or external agent. Therefore, this group faces a high risk of complications and death if they become infected with COVID-19.

Immunosuppressed patients include those affected by the Human Immunodeficiency Virus (HIV) and its consequent Acquired Immunodeficiency Syndrome (AIDS). In these people, the defense system is practically destroyed, facilitating the appearance of all kinds of bacterial, viral or fungal infections in the lungs and other organs.

People with diabetes can also have a weakened immune system. A special case to mention is the case of people with nutritional problems, either obesity or malnutrition, which generally see their body's ability to defend itself against infections reduced.

The group of cancer patients, who require immunosuppressive drugs, also shows a serious risk of complications and deaths when infected with COVID-19.

66. Mentally ill and disabled

The mentally ill are among the groups most vulnerable to contagion with COVID-19. Chinese authorities discovered in early February 2020 that many mental patients had acquired COVID-19 after being exposed to the infection because they were unable to consciously follow basic measures to avoid contact with sick people and contaminated objects.

Others suffered exposure to the virus in the psychiatric wards and institutions where they were detained, who in many cases did not have adequate sanitary measures to prevent an infection of this type.

A situation that affects the mentally ill is the stigma against them in the health system of many countries, which makes it difficult for them to receive timely care when they show symptoms of COVID-19.

To this is added that its treatment may require more attention and time from health personnel, which in many cases is already overwhelmed by cases of COVID-19 among the general population.

COVID-19 also causes a wave of fear and anxiety in society, which can aggravate the mental health of these patients, while quarantines and restrictions on the movement of people can affect compliance with the regular consultations and therapies they need.

Part VII. Global and community epidemiology

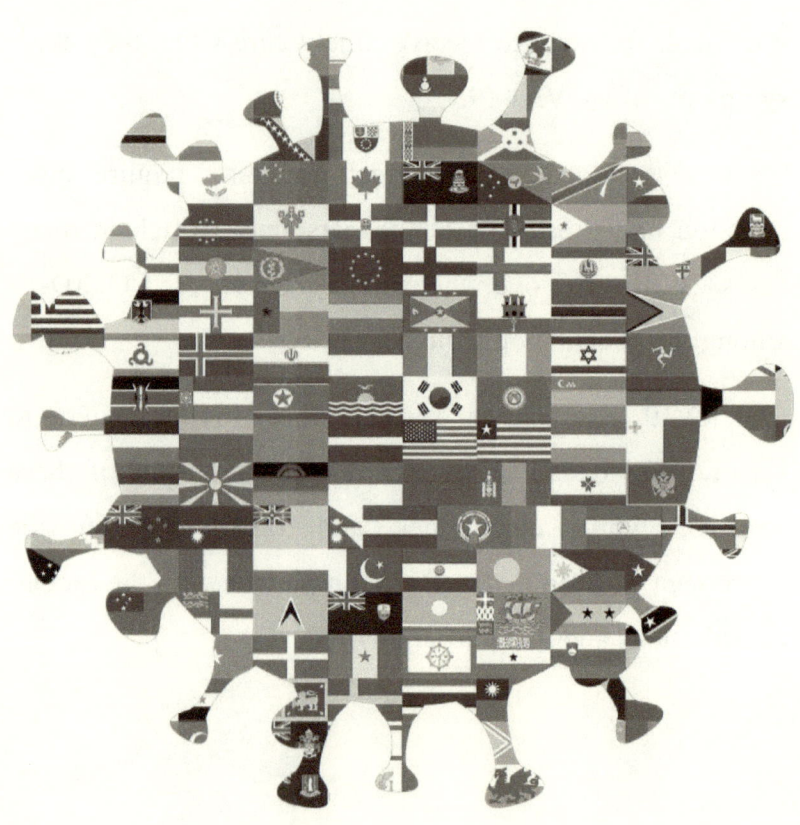

67. Epidemics in the history of humanity

Since Humanity keeps an oral or written record of its history, there have been a great number of epidemics that have killed millions of people in different regions of the world.

Many epidemics were caused by a single infectious agent and in others by a combination of two or more diseases, favored by poor hygiene conditions and poor diet among the population.

From 430 B.C. to the 21st century there have been 20 pandemics, or global or extra-continental epidemics. Among these, the four most destructive correspond to the epidemics of smallpox, Spanish flu, HIV-AIDS and the so-called black plague.

The smallpox epidemic is considered the most fatal in the entire history of Humanity, as well as the oldest, since this disease has raged for about 12,000 years. Since then more than 300 million men, women and children have died from the Poxvirus responsible for smallpox.

The most serious outbreak occurred between 1520 and 1533, when more than 56 million indigenous people from Central and South America died, infected by Spanish conquerors against whom they were fighting.

It was not until 1800 that a smallpox vaccine appeared, beginning a universal immunization plan that allowed the planet to be declared free of this disease in the late 1970s.

Measles is another disease characterized by causing deadly epidemics. It is estimated that since its appearance in ancient times, it has claimed more than 200 million victims. Until the invention of a vaccine in 1963, this disease appeared in cycles of 2 to 3 years, causing each time about 2 million deaths.

Another ancient and deadly epidemic that marked history was the Black Death, or bubonic plague, caused by the Yersinia pestis bacillus.

In the year 1347 a Black Death pandemic occurred that over the next 4 years killed 50 million Europeans and 150 million people in Asia and Africa. Overall, it is believed to have wiped out 42% of the world's population at the time.

The Yersinia pestis bacillus was transmitted by the bite of lice and fleas that reached Europe in the black rats that infested ships from China. His symptoms were swollen lymph nodes in the body and sexual organs, as well as pustules on the skin and necrosis of the limbs.

Another deadly pandemic that was recorded in recent history was the Spanish Flu of 1918. It was caused by a strain of the Influenza virus that emerged in Kansas, United States, and was brought to Europe by soldiers in the final stage of the First War. World. These infected soldiers arrived in France through the port of Brest and within a few weeks the outbreak spread to Great Britain, Germany, Italy and Spain.

Over the next 12 months, it killed 50 million lives in Europe and another 50 million in the United States and the rest of the world.

The name of the Spanish flu was due to the fact that the pandemic was widely discussed in this country and that it was not censored by the media, as it did in the other nations involved in World War I.

Before the recent COVID-19 pandemic, the one that caused the most fear in the world was the Human Immunodeficiency Virus (HIV), which appeared in the

United States in 1981. It is supposed to have originated in African monkeys and from there it spread to the humans.

This virus is transmitted by vaginal fluids and saliva during sexual contact, as well as by blood transfusions or by sharing contaminated needles among people addicted to drugs.

The infected mother can transmit HIV to the fetus in pregnancy or to the newborn during lactation. If it is not treated in time with retrovirals, its mortality rate is 80%.

Those infected develop Acquired Immune Deficiency Syndrome (AIDS), a destructive process of the immune system that exposes the patient to death from pneumonia and various infections.

From 1981 to the present, HIV-AIDS has killed about 35 million people and 37 million more are infected worldwide, according to the WHO.

68. Previous coronavirus epidemics

In 2003, the WHO issued a global alert on an epidemic of a new type of pneumonia that had appeared in the region of

Guangzhou, China. The disease was called Severe Acute Respiratory Syndrome (SARS), and a group of Chinese researchers identified a bat-related coronavirus as causing it.

This coronavirus was named SARS-CoV and although a rapid detection method could be developed, it was not possible to find a sufficiently effective medicine to counteract its action in the body.

SARS is characterized by causing severe pneumonia, fever above 38°C and severe organic complications, all in a relatively short period of time from the appearance of the first symptoms.

According to the WHO, the 2003 SARS outbreak affected 8,098 people in 24 countries around the world, of which 774 died. This gives a SARS-CoV case fatality rate of 9.6%.

On the other hand, in 2012 the appearance of a serious respiratory disease was reported in Saudi Arabia, which spread to Oman, Jordan and other countries in the Middle East through travelers. This was named Middle East Respiratory Syndrome (MERS) and a coronavirus linked to camels was identified as its cause, although later the contagion happened to be through direct personal contact.

This coronavirus was named MERS-CoV. Symptoms of MERS include high fever, dry cough, and shortness of breath.

From its appearance in 2012 to the present, MERS has killed 820 people and infected 2,357, representing a fatality rate of 34.8%.

69. Start, development and end of the pandemic

The pandemic begins the moment a disease spreads beyond one country and affects other nations and continents. The WHO has pointed out that pandemics are mainly related to infectious diseases caused by recently emerging viruses or bacteria, for which the population has no natural immunity.

Furthermore, the pandemic is favored by the late response of the health systems due to lack of equipment or due to the lack of an effective treatment or vaccine for the new disease.

The development of a pandemic is usually fast but short and its level of severity is not always rated just because of the number of deaths it causes.

In many cases the severity is in the thousands of patients that can arise in a short period of time, generating a serious public health problem.

For example, the Spanish flu pandemic was both rapid and lethal. In just 12 months, 50 million people died worldwide, more than the victims of World War I, which lasted 4 years.

Pandemics are terminated once new cases appear only in the same geographic area or country and do not transcend national borders.

70. Possibilities of local endemics

An endemic is defined as the regular appearance of a disease in the same region or country and in a similar number of cases in each cycle. Although a disease may also occur in other countries, it is considered to be endemic when it reappears continuously in the same geographical area and maintains a regular number of infected.

For example, malaria is an endemic disease in tropical countries and despite the controls and treatments applied by the different governments, it is estimated that each year it infects some 300 million people.

In the case of COVID-19, there are several studies underway to evaluate the possibility that SARS-CoV-2 acquires endemic qualities. Some cases of people who were reinfected after being discharged from South Korea and China, cast doubt on whether the population will develop a natural immunity against COVID-19 over time.

This suggests to some researchers that COVID-19 could reappear from time to time in the same place, becoming an endemic disease.

For this reason, it works to end the spread of the virus to a level that breaks its permanence within the same human group.

71. Local, national and international measures

In the framework of the COVID-19 pandemic, different measures of local, national and international scope can be applied to curb contagion.

At the local level, the most used are quarantines, social distancing and social isolation. Quarantine consists of the closure for several hours or permanently of families in their homes.

For its part, social distancing consists of a measure of separation of at least 1 meter between people who must go out to the streets to buy food or medicine, work or use public transportation.

Social isolation generally applies to those who become infected and must remain out of all contact, in their home or a designated space, for the duration of the infection.

At the national level, a widely used measure is the closure of transport between cities, as well as trains and flights that cover domestic routes.

The objective is to avoid the possible spread of contagion from one area of the country to another. During the pandemic in China, this measure was applied in Hubei province, with very good results.

At the international level, the most common measures against COVID-19 have been the closure of borders and the suspension of tourist flights or passenger transport by sea and land. The only exceptions applied have been to flights to repatriate foreign citizens and to the transport of cargo of medicines, food and basic supplies.

Another measure has been the installation of sanitary fences at border points to serve people entering each country and verify if they have symptoms of COVID-19.

72. Quarantine and social isolation

Among the non-medical measures most commonly applied by governments to curb the spread of a pandemic are quarantine and social isolation. In the case of viruses and coronaviruses, the basic objective of both measures is to cut the person-person transmission cycle by separating and isolating sick and healthy individuals.

This separation is for a time slightly longer than that required by the disease to manifest itself from the moment of infection. Both concepts may seem similar, but in reality they are two different things.

Social isolation consists of separating people with contagious diseases from healthy individuals. Most government health agencies point out that a socially isolated patient should not leave his home for the time indicated, nor receive visits. In addition, he should be confined to an area of the home separated from the rest of the family group.

For its part, quarantine is a measure of movement restriction for all those who may have been exposed to a contagion and are still asymptomatic for the minimum time required for said disease to manifest symptoms.

A quarantine is typically only mandated by national, state, or local health governing bodies when they want to slow down the spread of an infectious disease, whether it is an outbreak, an epidemic, or a pandemic.

Furthermore, it is also a useful tool to avoid large-scale infections that may exceed the capacity of hospital care in a country, region or city, especially if there are limitations in the supply of medicines and equipment.

In the framework of the COVID-19 pandemic, many governments ordered suspension of educational activities, collective meetings, cultural and sporting events, and even commercial and business activities.

WHO believes that social distancing and quarantine measures help to reduce the transmission chain of COVID-19, but only if they are accompanied by massive tests to rule out suspicious cases among the population, isolate confirmed cases, and trace and examine those have had contact with these.

73. Individual protection for the sick

The protection measures for COVID-19 patients are aimed both at preventing them from contracting other infections that worsen their condition, and at infecting other people in their environment.

The COVID-19 patient who is asymptomatic or with mild symptoms should be quarantined at home or in a specially conditioned place with good ventilation. If possible, you should use a bathroom that is different from the rest of the family, as well as bedding, towels, plates and cutlery.

These items should be washed with very hot water and whoever is in charge of this task should wear gloves and wash their hands as soon as they finish, even if they have been worn.

It is also important to clean frequently touched objects and surfaces every day, such as remote controls, door knobs, cell phones, light switches, kitchen tables and countertops.

When the patient is cared for by a caregiver, both should use a mask or cloth protection in their mouth and nose to reduce the emission of infected droplets into the air when speaking, breathing or coughing.

When coughing or sneezing, the COVID-19 patient should use a disposable tissue, which should be thrown away immediately and wash their hands with soap or antiseptic solution for at least 20 seconds.

COVID-19 patients who have previous conditions such as diabetes, heart failure, kidney or liver failure, must maintain strict compliance with the corresponding treatments.

They should not alter the doses of medicines without medical authorization and if their symptoms worsen they should immediately inform the emergency services to receive the necessary help. This includes situations such as the appearance of chest pain, respiratory failure, and a very high and continuous cough.

74. Individual protection of your contacts

The first step that every person infected with COVID-19 must do is report their situation to the people they have had contact with in the last 14 days at home, work and other places they have frequented.

People close to those infected by COVID-19 must take extreme hygiene and prevention measures. This includes avoiding physical contact with the patient and washing your hands several times a day with soapy solution or an alcohol-based antiseptic gel.

In the case of sharing the same home, a clear separation must be made of the space occupied by the patient and that used by the rest of the family group. This will help avoid exposure to contagion by touching contaminated surfaces or aspirating droplets emitted from the patient's breath.

If the patient shares the use of articles with the family, such as computers or telephones, these should be cleaned with a cloth and alcohol-based solution before others use them.

It is convenient for people close to a COVID-19 patient to apply a measure of self-isolation, especially during the first 14 days after the symptoms appeared.

If they have to go outside, they should wear a mask and gloves and keep a distance of at least 1 meter with other people.

75. Protection of the health professional

Medical and health personnel form the first line of battle against COVID-19 and are the work group most exposed to contagion.

In the first two months of the pandemic in China, Spain and Italy, up to 30% of hospital medical personnel had been infected with COVID-19 and many lost their lives.

The WHO has pointed out the extreme importance of guaranteeing health personnel the personal protection implements in the quantity and quality required to avoid contagion with SARS-CoV-2.

Studies carried out in Spain before the enormous percentage of doctors and nurses infected by COVID-19 indicated that the personal protective equipment used regularly in hospitals does not prevent SARS-CoV-2 from entering the respiratory tract and eyes of healthcare personnel.

After several modifications to the health protocols, it was recommended that medical personnel use integral protective equipment that includes medical masks, N95 or higher category respirators, face shields, gloves, gowns and closed suits.

However, it should be noted that SARS-CoV-2 has an average size of 120 nanometers or 0.12 microns, so N95 masks cannot prevent its entry into the user's airways.

For this reason, the use of P100 or R100 masks has been proposed, accompanied by a surgical mask inside and a face screen on the outside.

However, in the vast majority of countries it is impossible to supply these supplies to hospitals in the necessary quantity, which increased the exposure of health personnel to infection.

WHO Director-General Tedros Adhanom Ghebreyesus reported in early April that 89 million masks, 76 million gloves and 1.6 million safety glasses would be required each month to protect health personnel worldwide

The mental and psychological health of health personnel during the COVID-19 pandemic is also an issue to be addressed. These personnel are subjected to continuous stress and a huge workload, in addition to continually exposing themselves to traumatic situations in the death of large numbers of patients.

In addition, doctors, nurses, stretcher-bearers and even cleaning personnel in health centers can become sources of infection for their family and friends, if they become infected.

The WHO has also stressed the importance of governments protecting health personnel against social stigma by a public fearful of being a source of contagion.

In 2014, there was a history of assaults on doctors who fought the Ebola outbreak in West Africa.

In early April 2020, verbal and physical attacks were also reported against doctors and nurses in Colombia and Mexico, as they arrived at their homes after a long day of work caring for COVID-19 patients.

76. Protection of security personnel

In the framework of the COVID-19 pandemic, the security personnel responsible for guaranteeing the supply of protective equipment and supplies to health networks must also comply with the rules for the prevention of contagion.

The use of individual protection elements such as masks, gloves, full suits and others that prevent the entry of the coronavirus into your organisms is mandatory.

This is especially important among those working in COVID-19 designated patient care hospitals as well as in intensive care units.

Those responsible for security personnel who work outside hospitals must also have protection teams, that is, assisting those who carry out tasks to control vehicles and people or comply with sanitary measures in markets and food distribution centers during quarantines.

77. Declaration of cessation of quarantine

On April 8, the Chinese government declared the cessation of the collective quarantine in Wuhan, ordered 76 days before, being the first country to lift a quarantine measure in the framework of the COVID-19 pandemic.

This decision was made after several days without registering new deaths from COVID-19 throughout the Chinese mainland.

Furthermore, only 271 cases of infection were recorded, mainly in Chinese citizens who returned from abroad.

Quarantining in Wuhan was key to preventing the virus from spreading to the rest of mainland China. To date, 3,331 people have died in the country, of whom 2,571 were residents of Wuhan. There were also 81,700 infected, of which 50,008 corresponded to inhabitants of this city.

After declaring the cessation of quarantine, the Hubei province government reported that only citizens with a special certificate guaranteeing their good health and who have had no contact with people suspected of having COVID would be allowed to travel to other regions. 19.

The WHO has indicated that quarantine measures should aim to break the COVID-19 cycle of person-to-person transmission, so its suspension in any city or country will depend on how much the numbers of new infections and deaths drop.

78. Declaration of cessation of transmission

The WHO has recommended that COVID-19 declarations of cessation of transmission be made only when 14 days have elapsed without new cases. This is the average time it takes for symptoms to appear and is a reference used for the isolation of suspicious cases.

79. Notifiable disease

Due to the high rate of contagion and risk of death represented by COVID-19, the vast majority of governments declared the obligation to report any suspected case, as well as the subsequent confirmation and evolutionary follow-up of the patients.

In addition, citizens traveling or living in countries where cases have been reported are required to report to the authorities if they have any symptoms.

Private clinics, hospitals and private doctors are obliged to inform health authorities about any patient with symptoms of dry cough, shortness of breath and to inform the authorities, who will apply the respective epidemiological surveillance strategy.

Part VIII. Prevention of disease

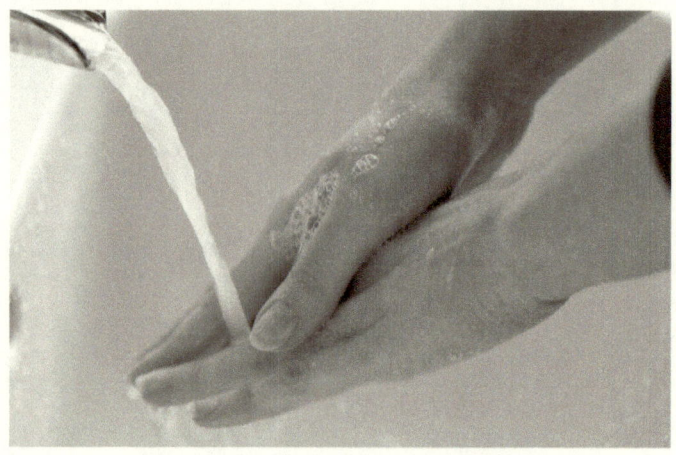

80. Surveillance for symptom-free contacts

One of the most important measures to stop the COVID-19 pandemic is to cut the SARS-CoV-2 transmission cycle from person to person. For this, those who have had contact with confirmed COVID-19 patients must be identified and monitored.

According to the protocols established by the WHO, confirmed cases with mild or asymptomatic symptoms should be cared for at home, in conditions of quarantine and social isolation.

On the other hand, moderate to severe cases must be attended in health centers. But the contacts of confirmed COVID-19 patients should also be located and attended as soon as possible.

Contacts are defined as any person who has shared with the COVID-19 patient a common workspace, home, social gathering, or used the same equipment or supplies. A distinction is made between close contact and casual contact. The first refers to family group members and coworkers or friends who have been less than 2 meters away from a person with symptoms for a long time.

For its part, the term casual contact refers to people who share the same physical space as the infected with COVID-19 but do not maintain physical contact or closeness to it, such as coworkers who are in other areas of the company or neighbors of a building.

The classification of this type of contact is at the discretion of the epidemiological surveillance services, but the clinical follow-up will be done only for close contacts. Close contacts that show no symptoms should be quarantined for 14 days in a fixed location.

Rapid diagnostic tests have begun to be applied to these contacts in some countries and not in others. You should measure your temperature twice a day and notify the health authorities if a symptom appears such as fever greater than 38°C, cough and difficulty breathing.

Once the 14 days of quarantine have passed without manifestation of symptoms, the epidemiological surveillance of the contact is terminated.

81. Caring for the patient with COVID-19 at home

In most cases, COVID-19 patients will only show mild symptoms and will be advised to rest at home. The care you receive at home is intended to keep symptoms from complicating and to protect other family members from infection.

This is especially important if the patient lives with adults over the age of 60 or other family members suffering from underlying diseases such as diabetes, heart disease or some type of lung disease. It is also true if the person who meets these conditions is the caregiver of a patient with COVID-19.

The COVID-19 patient must stay home and comply with a strict quarantine of at least 14 days, after which they must be evaluated by doctors to certify if the infection has ceased.

The patient should be isolated in a room separated from the rest of the family, sufficiently ventilated and, if possible, use a bathroom only for him. Patients with COVID-19 cannot share personal or kitchen utensils, bedding, or personal clothing with other family members.

A minimum distance of 2 meters must be maintained with the rest of the inhabitants of the home.

It is important to clean the surfaces of the bathroom and bathroom furniture used by the patient, with a disinfecting solution based on sodium hypochlorite or alcohol. Light switches, kitchen counters, and door handles should also be disinfected.

The use of the mask by the infected is essential. This mask must be changed daily. They must also be used by those who enter the patient's room to care for him.

If the patient cannot wear a mask, the mouth and nose should be covered with disposable tissues when sneezing or coughing, and thrown away immediately.

The caregiver of the patient with COVID-19 should wear gloves when handling the clothing, and avoid at all costs direct contact with body fluids such as feces, urine or mucus. Both gloves and masks used in patient care should be thrown away as soon as they are finished using.

The entire family group should wash their hands several times a day with disinfectant gel or an alcohol-based solution in a concentration equal to or greater than 60%.

82. Transfer of suspects or sick

The transfer of a suspected or confirmed patient with COVID-19 requires certain considerations that must be fulfilled by the medical transport and pre-hospital care services.

These considerations aim to reduce the risk of contagion for the personnel in charge of the ambulances, as well as other patients who use them later.

Before starting the care transfer operation of a suspected or confirmed patient with COVID-19, their needs for stabilization should be taken into account, such as assisted breathing equipment, serums and medications.

Patients who receive assisted breathing should be transferred to their own bed, to avoid contamination risks when disconnecting tubes and accessories in ambulances.

Disposable costumes, masks, face shields, gloves, and all available protective equipment must be used by transfer personnel and must be discarded upon delivery to the patient.

Then you must put on new personal protective equipment and proceed to disinfect the ambulance and all used equipment.

83. Complicated hospitalization

In general, patients with COVID-19 show mild or moderate symptoms such as fever of 38°C, and cough, so the medical measure applied is rest at home for at least 2 weeks, while the infection subsides.

However, when symptoms worsen and shortness of breath, chest pain, cardiac arrhythmia, high blood pressure, and other problems appear, immediate hospitalization of the patient is urgent.

In this case, the patient complicated with COVID-19 should be placed in an isolated single room or a space dedicated only to patients with this disease.

Visits should be restricted or prohibited if necessary and all who enter these rooms must use adequate protection.

Whenever possible, the transfer of a patient complicated with COVID-19 between different areas of the health center should be avoided. Should additional studies be required, such as ultrasound and X-rays, efforts should be made to do so with portable equipment in the patient's room.

If the hospital equipment is not mobile, it must be fully disinfected once used by the patient with COVID-19.

In the hospitalization of complicated cases with COVID-19, the priority of the treating team is to preserve respiratory function and attend to complications that may occur at the liver, coronary or renal level.

The availability of assisted ventilation equipment in key when deciding the hospitalization of a patient with COVID-19 that shows severe or complicated symptoms.

84. Short-term hospitalization centers

Short-term hospitalization centers offer a timely solution to the overflow of health services due to the high volume of suspected patients with COVID-19. In areas where the pandemic has left a large number of infected and victims, the use of provisional hospital centers has been used, aimed solely at the care of patients with COVID-19.

Additionally, many hospitals in countries such as China, Spain, Italy, the United States and Germany have closed their different services to dedicate all their physical space to patients with COVID-19.

The creation of field hospitals, sometimes in rare places like New York's Central Park, is part of the response to the collapse of formal health centers.

These short-term hospitalization centers have the advantage of having the necessary equipment to care for patients with COVID-19 and its possible complications.

This includes X-ray and digital imaging equipment, intensive care units, mechanical ventilators and everything necessary to manage a highly contagious patient at high risk.

85. Intensive care and assisted ventilation

When a COVID-19 patient develops severe symptoms, the most obvious and most life-threatening is acute respiratory distress syndrome (ARDS).

This syndrome occurs due to obstruction with very thick phlegm of the alveoli and bronchi. A severe patient with COVID-19 is considered to lose up to 70 percent of his lung capacity due to phlegm and injury to his lung lobes.

Both in patients who were healthy before becoming infected with COVID-19, and in those who had previous conditions such as heart disease, hypertension, diabetes and others, loss of respiratory capacity is always the greatest danger they face.

For this reason, severe cases should be treated with assisted breathing 24 hours a day during the phase in which symptoms of pneumonia and ARDS appear.

Intensive care is also required to care for complications in the cardiovascular system caused by low blood oxygen and inflammation of the vessels around the lungs and heart.

Kidney and liver failure are other common problems in severe cases with COVID-19, which also lead many patients to intensive care units.

86. General and immunological support measures

Patients with COVID-19 usually present with fever and cough during the initial phase of the disease. For this reason, your initial care should include continuous hydration to replenish electrolyte levels in the blood and help the phlegm that forms in the lungs to be expelled more easily.

In the case of patients with diseases that affect their defenses, doctors may evaluate therapies aimed at increasing their immune response, such as the use of interferon or treatments used successfully in cases of SARS and MERS.

At the moment, a particularly reliable drug has not been found to increase the immune response in uninfected patients and protect them from COVID-19.

However, studies are being done to determine the effectiveness of vitamin-based therapies and certain medications that stimulate the body's immune system.

87. Antivirals, antibiotics, and steroids

Although an effective treatment for SARS-CoV-2 has not yet been discovered, various universities and research groups are working to determine the usefulness of antivirals and medications used with relative success in other coronavirus diseases.

The use of antivirals is based on the fact that SARS-CoV-2 belongs to the Betacoronavirus group, which also includes SARS-CoV and MERS-CoV, causing Middle East Respiratory Syndrome (MERS).

Some Ebola medications are also being tested to verify their action against SARS-CoV-2.

Interferon is currently used by China, Cuba and other countries as part of the treatment of patients in their initial stages, with good results.

The efficacy of drugs such as ribavirin, lopinavir-ritonavir, and penciclovir, remdesivir, and favipiravir are also being tested, which are showing a significant effect of reducing the viral load in the blood of those infected.

As for corticosteroids, their use is applied in certain conditions where inflammation of the lung tissues can cause permanent damage or a collapse of respiratory function.

So far, several governments are promoting the use of Chloroquine and its variants, used in the treatment of malaria, as a way to reduce the viral load of SARS-CoV-2.

Although the use of chloroquine is not yet supported in clinical studies related to COVID-19, many cases of improvement have been reported in moderate to severe patients receiving this drug.

One possible reason is that chloroquine increases endosomal pH, which affects the process of fusion of the virus with human cells. It also has an immunomodulatory effect and its efficiency seems the same both in initial and advanced stages of infection.

The application of antibiotics in patients with COVID-19 aims to attack secondary infections with pneumococci and other bacteria in those who have developed sepsis or septic shock.

88. Current and future vaccines

Several countries are working on a vaccine against COVID-19, applying information on the SARS-CoV-2 genome released by Chinese scientists investigating the pandemic in Wuhan, Hubei province.

For the most part, these synthetic vaccines use a genetic code that instructs human cells to produce a protein present in SARS-CoV-2, used to gain entry into cells.

In this way, the body generates an immune response to that protein and therefore, the ability of the causative agent of COVID-19 to invade human cells is reduced.

However, in the best case, the first one will only complete the experimentation and certification steps towards the last quarter of 2020.

Researchers from at least five countries are working to verify theories that current vaccines, such as the Bacille Calmette-Guerin (BCG) or the tuberculosis vaccine, increase the body's ability to defend itself against COVID-19.

This is based on evidence found in previous experiences and studies that suggests that BCG "trains" the immune system to recognize and react not only to the Koch bacillus, but also to a wide variety of bacteria, parasites and viruses.

According to one of the ongoing studies based on the case of 150,000 children vaccinated with BCG in 33 countries, these had 40% of acute respiratory infections than the unvaccinated.

A similar relationship was also found in the case of older adults, who suffered fewer respiratory infections than unvaccinated children.

89. Chronically ill control

Chronic patients should be extremely careful in case of getting COVID-19, especially if they suffer from illnesses or receive treatments that affect the immune system.

The first step is to stay in quarantine or isolation at home and not expose yourself to contagion when shopping. These tasks need to be delegated to someone you trust.

Chronic patients affected by COVID-19 who have not developed symptoms that warrant hospitalization should continue with their regular treatments and not alter them without medical authorization.

In the case of diabetic patients, it is recommended to monitor glucose levels, as well as body temperature, at least three times a day.

Hypertensive and cardiovascular patients should maintain rest and check their blood pressure twice a day, especially if there are signs of respiratory distress or signs of pneumonia, a condition that can affect cardiac oxygenation.

In the case of patients with respiratory diseases such as emphysema, tuberculosis and asthma, it is recommended that they be placed in hospital care immediately, as they are a group with a high risk of complications and mortality from COVID-19.

90. Vitamins and nutrition

There are several trials and studies underway to assess the impact of vitamin insufficiency on the body's vulnerability to COVID-19 infection. However, these studies have so far not been categorical and for the most part build on previous experiences with other diseases caused by viruses such as dengue and influenza.

Several studies seem to point out that a boost in oral vitamin D consumption seems to help reduce the severity of respiratory symptoms in patients complicated with COVID-19.

This seems to be related to the capacity of vitamin D as an anti-inflammatory in lung tissues, as well as the fact that the coronavirus and the influenza or influenza virus share common characteristics.

Among these, they highlight that both viruses are capped with the capacity to survive outside a host and their mortality is mainly related to severe pneumonia.

The possible relationship between poor exposure to sunlight, vital for the synthesis of vitamin D in the body, with the large number of cases of COVID-19 registered among the populations of China, South Korea and Europe is also studied.

This study also finds that Africa and South America, where sun exposure is highest, appear to have a much slower rate of infection.

The studies propose a substantial increase in the intake of vitamin D, of more than 5,000 IU daily in the case of people younger than 50 years.

In the case of adults over 50 years of age in serious condition, the intake of 10,000 IU per day or up to 100,000 per week is proposed, for as long as the symptoms of the disease persist.

Regarding vitamin C, traditionally related to the proper functioning of the immune system, there have been no indications that an increase in its consumption protects the body against COVID-19.

This has been verified in critically ill patients who received high doses of vitamin C intravenously, without major variation in their clinical state.

The theoretical value of vitamin C as therapy for COVID-19 patients is based on a 2017 study that found a substantial reduction in deaths in patients with sepsis who were administered a high amount of vitamin C combined with corticosteroids and thiamine.

In 2019, it was found that patients with acute respiratory distress syndrome (ARDS) found improvement with a treatment with a high concentration of vitamin C.

In China, a study is being carried out regarding this vitamin and COVID-19, the results of which could be ready by September 2020.

91. Management of social and individual stress

The COVID-19 pandemic has caused widespread fear among societies in practically every country in the world, especially with those with the highest number of infected and deaths, such as China, Italy, Spain, France and the United States.

Social isolation and restrictions on individual mobility during the pandemic have also contributed to increasing the level of stress in population groups and individuals.

The main concerns of the population are the economic issue due to the closure of thousands of companies and activities on which many families depend.

Also the alteration of daily routines and the fear of contracting the disease cause a great emotional charge in people.

Added to this is the uncertainty about the duration of the pandemic and what permanent or lasting changes it will leave in society when it reaches its end. Also contributing to collective stress is the excess of information, often confusing or contradictory, about this pandemic, in social networks and the media.

In this regard, the WHO has recommended governments and the media to work in campaigns to guide the population in the emotional management of quarantine.

This includes promoting self-care measures such as getting enough sleep, exercising at home, or doing some physical activity that helps drain tension and improve mood. Eating healthy and avoiding excess sugar, coffee, and salt are also encouraged.

The campaigns also call for avoiding the consumption of drugs, alcohol and tobacco, as these increase the body's vulnerability to COVID-19.

An important measure is to reduce exposure to the internet and TV, as well as to social networks that expose false information about the pandemic.

92. Natural and traditional treatments

In the framework of the fight against COVID-19, the Chinese authorities allowed the use of some traditional treatments in moderate and severe patients, with good results.

The pharmaceutical company Shijiashazhuang Yiling patented a medicine in capsules called Lianhua Qingwen (LHQW), based on Traditional Chinese Medicine (MTC), which, combined with western medicines, gave good results by decreasing the intensity of symptoms.

This drug had already been successfully tested during the 2003 SARS pandemic, which appeared in China and spread to some 24 countries.

Clinical trials indicate that LHQW relieves respiratory symptoms such as dry cough, cough with phlegm, and respiratory distress. It also helps reduce the duration of fever and the intensity of dyspnea. It is currently used in Chinese clinics and hospitals in moderate and severe COVID-19 patients.

Following the Chinese experience, in early April 2020 countries such as Italy, Venezuela and Ecuador authorized the use of this medicine in patients with COVID-19.

It previously had authorization from the governments of Romania, Macao, Thailand, Canada, Mozambique, Indonesia and Brazil, some of which used it in the 2003 SARS epidemic.

Another traditional medicine that is used in the fight against COVID-19 is a 20-plant based cooking used in China as a detoxifier and for cleaning the lungs, called "Quing Fei Jie Du Tang". This cooking includes both oriental plants such as mandarin, almond, ephedra, ginger and coriander.

The General Office of the National Health Committee and the Office of the State Administration of Traditional Chinese Medicine recommend this cooking to hospitals that care for patients with COVID-19.

Part IX. Individual and collective protection

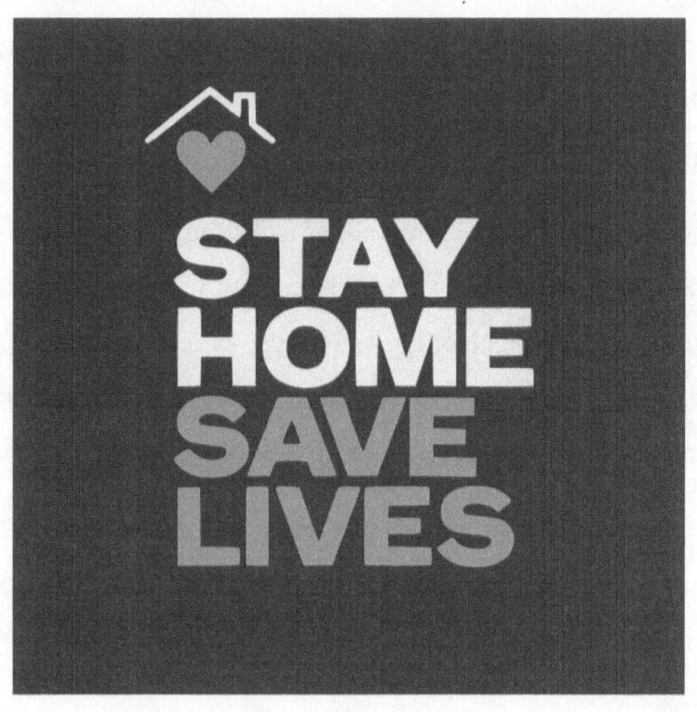

93. Weather care

So far, no clear relationship has been found between the climate and the contagion capacity of COVID-19. Various studies indicate that SARS-CoV-2 can easily withstand ambient temperatures of 38° C and others indicate that it can survive for two hours at temperatures up to 60° C.

Where there does seem to be a relationship is in the level of exposure to sunlight, which favors those who live in tropical areas against contagion.

In this regard, the WHO has indicated that the care for patients with COVID-19 and the general population with respect to the climate are the same as those applied for other diseases such as influenza and influenza.

Those who live in cold climates should try to stay warm at all times and not expose themselves to extreme cold or icy baths, as a precaution.

For their part, those who live in tropical climates or in areas with high summer temperatures are recommended to maintain constant hydration and take care not to overexpose themselves to the sun.

94. Use and type of masks

The masks or face shields used in the framework of the COVID-19 pandemic should cover two main functions: to protect health personnel who care for potential infected or confirmed infections and to protect healthy people in their normal work or home environments.

The majority of the population should wear surgical masks when going outside, using public transport or doing any activity outside in places where there is a crowding or presence of other people.

Surgical masks are so-called face masks used by doctors and nurses in surgeries and other health activities. They do not filter the inhaled air, so they cannot prevent the entry of nasal droplets expelled by infected people. However, they can protect against splashes of blood, mucus and other fluids from these people.

In addition, when a COVID-19 patient wears a mask, the number of droplets that go into the air when they breathe or cough is greatly reduced.

For this reason and because many people can be infected and not yet show symptoms, it is important that everyone wear surgical masks when going out on the street or having contact with other people at home or work.

Another type of masks very useful in the COVID-19 pandemic are those of the filter type, which contain a filter capable of closing the passage to liquid or solid microparticles present in the air. They are manufactured in different types and are classified according to the size of the particles that can be filtered. Its filtering efficiency of incoming particles ranging from 78% (FFPP1) to 98% (FFP3).

These filters also have a high capacity for filtering outgoing particles when breathing and coughing, with leak rates of 22% in FFP1 masks up to only 2% in FFP3 type ones.

Filtering masks of category FFP2 and FFP3 are considered to be the most efficient in preventing infection with COVID-19. Currently one of the most used masks worldwide is the N95 type, with filter and outlet valve to avoid condensation.

However, considering that the SARS-CoV-2 coronavirus can be up to 120 microns in size, some experts recommend the P100 and P200 models, which can filter out microparticles as low as 80 microns.

95. Hand washes

Handwashing is one of the recommendations that the WHO and the health entities of the countries with the highest number of COVID-19 infected have made with the most emphasis.

This practice is especially important because it has been found that the SAR-CoV-2 coronavirus can subsist for many hours on most materials for mass use in cities, such as glass, aluminum, steel, fabrics, paper, leather and latex.

To prevent contagion by touching potentially infected surfaces from contact with body fluids from a COVID-19 infection, it is recommended to wash your hands several times a day with plenty of soap and hot water.

It is important to rub all the spaces between the fingers, under the nails and the back of the hands for not less than 30 seconds and rinse with plenty of water. Also, they should be dried with a clean single-use towel or a disposable tissue.

Handwashing should also be done after blowing your nose, sneezing, or coughing, as well as each time you return from the street, using public transportation, or a public gathering place such as markets and churches. It is also recommended to do so if cash has been tampered with.

Those who care for a patient with COVID-19 or who is suspected of being infected should take extreme care in hand washing, as well as wearing masks and gloves.

96. Alcohol and antibacterial

Alcohol at a concentration of 60% or higher has been found to be effective in destroying the coronavirus causing COVID-19.

In this regard, the WHO recommends disinfecting with concentrated alcohol the objects and surfaces with which people have the most contact in homes and public spaces.

For the disinfection of surfaces such as streets, walls, vehicles and large urban areas, it is recommended to use a solution based on sodium hypochlorite or some antibacterial disinfectant for industrial use.

Regarding the use of antibacterial gel, the Centers for Disease Control of the United States and the governing bodies of health of the European Union agree that these are only useful as a measure of temporary disinfection when you cannot wash your hands with soap and water.

This is a situation that frequently occurs in regions of the planet where drinking water service is irregular or does not exist. In this case, it is recommended to use antibacterial gel that has a concentrated alcohol base of at least 60 to 70%.

It is recommended is to apply abundant gel on the palms of the hands and rub them for at least 20 seconds, trying to spread the gel between the fingers, under the nails and on the back of the hand.

97. Lifestyle, exercise and mental health

Maintaining a healthy lifestyle helps the body stay fit and therefore increases its ability to resist a viral infection like COVID-19. In the context of quarantine applied in many countries, millions of people have had to stay for days at home, thus reducing their daily activity and boredom and other forms of stress due to the change in normal routine.

During quarantine it is important to distribute the schedule to maintain some type of activity that allows you to distract the mind and keep the body in shape.

Reading books, learning languages, watching series and movies, or trying to learn a new hobby are some of the recommendations made by psychologists and behavioral experts to those who are quarantined.

Likewise, it is recommended to maintain a complete diet and perform some type of exercise. It is important to avoid falling into an excessive consumption of fats and sugars, which in combination with sedentary lifestyle can have serious consequences such as changes in blood glucose.

Family life can be affected by long isolation, so it is recommended to do shared activities such as games, clean the house or practice some kind of hobby among several, in order to avoid conflicts during this time.

98. Ventilation of houses and rooms

Ventilation of houses and spaces where people infected with COVID-19 are housed is essential to avoid the concentration of the virus in the air.

The patient's room should have continuous ventilation or at least be ventilated 4 times a day, as recommended by the United States Centers for Disease Control.

The United States Environmental Protection Agency (EPA) has pointed out that inside a house closed to the outside, as occurs in the most intense winters and summers, the concentration of polluting elements can exceed up to 100 times that of the outside air.

These pollutants include smoke from stoves and ovens, carbon monoxide produced by gas cookers and heaters, and others such as nitrogen oxide and sulfur.

Other elements that are removed with adequate ventilation are mold, excess moisture, pet hair, oil particles and cooked food and dust.

For this reason, ventilation of homes and patient rooms with COVID-19 is recommended to reduce the load of pollutants in the air that could aggravate cough or respiratory distress in these patients. Furthermore, frequent ventilation of these spaces prevents characteristic symptoms of carbon dioxide accumulation, such as headaches and a drop in metabolism.

99. Homes for the elderly and disabled

One of the main public health problems that the COVID-19 pandemic has brought is the large number of deaths of older adults found in nursing homes.

In countries such as Great Britain and Spain the numbers of deceased elderly in these homes grow day by day and in many cases it has been discovered that caregivers have left them alone in the midst of quarantine.

People over the age of 60 are the group most likely to develop complications from a COVID-19 infection, so it is urgent to give them the greatest possible protection. This includes the supply of masks in sufficient quantities and the restriction of visits by family and friends, to reduce exposure to the coronavirus.

It is also important to follow up with those who have underlying medical conditions such as diabetes, hypertension, respiratory failure, or heart failure.

For their part, people with disabilities face a variety of challenges in the midst of the pandemic. Those affected by mental disabilities often have trouble communicating when they feel ill or explaining their symptoms to healthcare personnel.

They can also see their problems aggravated by the anxiety produced by the pandemic, social isolation and the change in their daily habits.

The restriction to move, product of the social quarantines imposed in many countries, can directly threaten the continuity of their treatments and therapies.

For their part, the physically handicapped face the same risks as the rest of the population when infected with COVID-19, except in cases where there are complications that affect their renal, hepatic, cardiovascular or respiratory systems.

Health agencies must ensure that these people have access to the therapies and treatments they need and closely monitor their health status in anticipation of any signs that they have been infected with COVID-19.

100. Markets and supermarkets

In the midst of the social quarantine implemented worldwide by the COVID-19 pandemic, food markets and distribution centers have continued to function as a priority sector for the population.

The risk of contagion in these places increases as the presence of a greater number of people close to each other is allowed.

For this reason, the WHO has issued protocols that advise that only a limited number of people enter these shops at a time, keeping a distance of at least 2 meters from one another and always wearing a mask and gloves.

Markets and supermarkets are regularly places where the cultivation of bacteria and pathogens is favored by the large number of organic and perishable products sold there.

In the framework of the pandemic, local, regional and national health entities have been instructed to carry out regular disinfection of these with solutions based on sodium hypochlorite and high concentration alcohol.

Continuous disinfection of surfaces such as counters, refrigerator doors, boxes, shelves and any item or furniture that may be touched by the public at any time must also be ensured.

Markets and supermarkets must, for reasons of collective interest, implement a home delivery service, to ensure the supply of food to the population without exposing them to possible contagion.

101. Restaurants and dining rooms

Depending on the country, the restaurants, canteens and shops that prepare meals may or may not be considered among the priority sectors that can continue to operate in the midst of the quarantine due to the COVID-19 pandemic.

However, in most countries restrictions have been applied to the operation of these venues, since they favor the congregation of a number of public that can exceed in many cases 15 people at a time.

As in the case of supermarkets and groceries, in many countries the authorities have urged restaurants to implement home delivery services, as a way to avoid exposing people to COVID-19.

102. Cinemas and theaters

The operation of cinemas, theaters and places of mass entertainment must be totally prohibited in the context of the fight against the COVID-19 pandemic. These places concentrate large numbers of people in a small space, which favors contagion.

In practically all countries that have quarantined due to COVID-19, regulations have been issued ordering the closure of this type of entertainment site.

The WHO has emphasized that any entertainment site where the public crowds is a potential focus of risk of spread of the SARS-CoV-2 coronavirus.

Therefore, he has stressed the call to the authorities not to favor their continued operation until the end of the pandemic is declared.

103. Lifts and stairs

It is recommended to avoid the use of elevators during the COVID-19 pandemic, since they are small spaces where a significant viral load can be concentrated if used by a sick person who is not properly protected with a mask and gloves.

Although the elevators have ventilation systems, in the vast majority of cases the air flow they produce is insufficient to quickly renew the fresh air.

In this way, the droplets emitted by a patient when breathing or coughing can be kept for a long period of time suspended inside the elevators.

An elevator's keypad or control panel is another potential source of infection if it is used by a sick person whose hands are contaminated with the virus.

In buildings where its use is unavoidable, the WHO recommends limiting the number of people boarding elevators to that which allows a distance of 1 meter to keep each other.

It is also recommended to disinfect your internal surfaces, especially the control panels and call buttons on each floor, several times a day with solutions based on concentrated alcohol.

In the case of ladders, both manual and mechanical, the priority is to disinfect the handrails as many times as possible and maintain a distance of 2 meters between one user and another.

104. Public and private transportation

Public transport is one of the systems that requires the most attention from health authorities, due to the fact that it is used by a large number of people at the same time.

In places where total quarantine has been declared, public transportation has been temporarily suspended, including intercity trains, subways, buses, and taxi services. In cities that do not yet restrict the use of buses and subways, health authorities have recommended reducing the volume of passengers per car or unit, in order to maintain adequate personal separation.

It has also been recommended to implement disinfection systems for wagons, buses, taxis and any other vehicle used as a means of mass transportation.

For its part, the use of private transport remains a safe way of moving in the midst of the pandemic, as long as its use does not violate the restrictions on the transit of people and vehicles during the quarantine.

105. Flights and airports

Air transport proved to be the main route of diffusion of COVID-19 from China to the rest of the world.

Following the appearance of the first COVID-19 outbreak in Wuhan, China, between the end of December 2019 and January 2020, many countries dismissed the first recommendations by scientists and researchers to limit or suspend flights to and from China. This encouraged thousands of people, both healthy and infected with or without symptoms, to travel from one continent to another.

The first cases recorded outside of China, in South Korea, Japan, Italy and other countries, were generally of people who had traveled to Wuhan and returned by plane. The first case in the United States was also of a person who had returned by air from China.

Airports are perhaps the biggest health problem that governments face to control the arrival of COVID-19 to their territories, as it happened with previous pandemics such as AH1N1 and SARS. In these facilities large numbers of people gather for hours in closed spaces, which is a permanent source of contagion.

Currently most countries in Europe, Latin America and the United States maintain a closure of international flights, with the exception of those aimed at repatriating stranded citizens in other countries.

If for some reason you must take a flight, it is important to wear protective equipment such as a mask, face shield, gloves and a protective suit, as well as check body temperature and vital signs.

In addition, at airports that maintain operations for the repatriation of nationals or the transport of medicines and cargo, rapid tests must be applied to the crew and passengers of the aircraft and the quarantine areas of travelers stranded by the closure of borders must be established.

106. Ports and cruises

Tourism cruises pose a high risk of contagion from viral and bacterial diseases, for various reasons. Added to the massive concentration of passengers, even thousands in some modern ships, is the fact that its interior is a kind of closed ecosystem where the air potentially contaminated with viruses and pathogens recirculates through dozens of cabins, rooms and decks before of being renovated from the outside.

In the framework of the COVID-19 pandemic, several cases of luxury cruises were reported in Asia, Europe and the United States where the presence of infected passengers was reported, many of them after visiting China and other Asian countries.

In most cases, passengers could not be disembarked for medical attention, due to the refusal of different governments to allow these ships to dock at their ports. This led to the death of many of the sick passengers, mainly the older ones.

Cruise travel is currently practically prohibited for health reasons and in light of the experience experienced at the start of the pandemic. The ports of loading and unloading are also nerve centers from the epidemiological point of view.

During the peak of the contagion chain in China, all tourist and commercial port operations were closed and were only reopened to a limited extent as the number of new cases fell in mid-April.

However, many import-dependent developing countries cannot take these types of port closure measures because these are their only route of entry for food and basic products.

In these cases, the WHO has recommended implementing sanitary customs for the inspection of crews and the disinfection of equipment and cargo arriving on board ships.

People who must travel by ship undergo a strict screening before boarding and must meet a quarantine period upon arrival.

107. Schools and Universities

The educational sector is another key point in the health prevention of COVID-19, which is why practically by mid-March all the countries of the world had ordered the suspension of classes from the initial level to the university level.

The WHO has emphasized the importance of this, because although adults over 60 years of age have a higher risk of complications from COVID-19, young people have the same possibilities of being infected as an older adult.

In addition, deaths of young people from a few months of age to 18 years have been reported and many of those infected are in the range of 25 to 49 years.

The availability of the internet and electronic resources for information management allow the education of children and young people to continue at home, through virtual classes and online learning.

In the framework of the COVID-19 pandemic, more than 130 countries implemented a suspension of face-to-face classes and its continuation through virtual classrooms or electronically.

In this way, the continuity and completion of the regular periods of primary and secondary education are guaranteed, as well as the advancement of undergraduate and postgraduate university courses.

In this sense, the WHO has recommended that countries that do not yet implement online classes to look for alternatives that allow the education of children and young people to continue in their homes and avoid exposing them to massive contagion if they attend schools and universities during the pandemic.

Part X. Summary of facts and clinical controversies

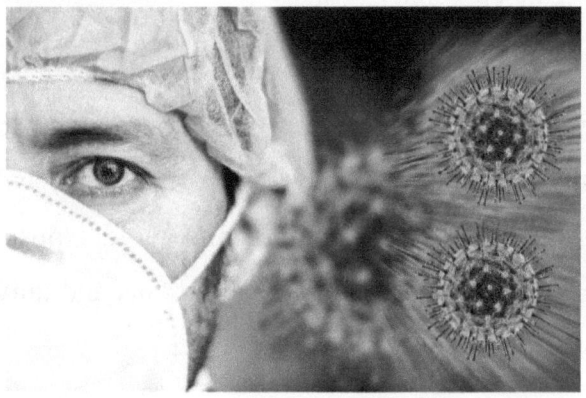

In this last part of the second volume of the book, the author is dedicated to clarifying some controversial points about clinical evolution, diagnosis, treatment and prevention measures, to complement all the information already exposed.

The book closes with a vision of the possible perspectives for the future of the world after controlling SARS-CoV-2 infection and COVID-19 disease

108. Explanations on COVID-19

Handwashing with soap, sodium hypochlorite, and antiseptic alcohol removes the virus

These three methods are effective in removing the virus, as long as they are applied well. In the case of hands, the washing should be for at least 30 seconds, rubbing the back and the spaces between the fingers well.

Sodium hypochlorite is very useful to sterilize potentially contaminated surfaces by contact of an infected person. In the case of antiseptic alcohol, it is only effective if its concentration is greater than 60%, it is capable of inactivating the virus after 1 minute.

Quarantine, social distancing and the use of masks will avoid infecting us

COVID-19 infection occurs when the nasal droplets emitted by a patient when coughing, breathing, or sneezing reach the mucous membranes (nose, mouth, conjunctiva) of a healthy person.

Although they seem simple, these three measures used together are very useful to reduce the possibility of contagion by cutting the person-to-person transmission cycle of SARS-CoV-2.

The most useful of the masks is that they stop a large part of the droplets with viral load expelled by infected people, whether or not they have symptoms of COVID-19. Social distance and quarantine in suspected cases notably help slow the spread of infections between groups of people, very important in populated centers and large cities.

Those infected without symptoms can transmit SARS-CoV-2

A small percentage of people infected with SARS-CoV-2 do not develop or take longer to show visible symptoms of the disease. However, they can spread to other people nearby through respiratory droplets that the infected expels when speaking, breathing or sneezing.

Some studies have concluded that an infected person can transmit the disease to others between 2 to 5 days before showing any symptoms. Furthermore, it was found that the viral load of these asymptomatic patients is similar to that of patients with mild or moderate symptoms.

It is a simple flu that attacks older people with low defenses

Statistics collected in China and Spain, countries heavily affected by the pandemic, indicate that the highest number of infected were located in the age range between 20 and 79 years of age, with a very low infection rate among those 0 to 19 years. Therefore, it is considered that SARS-CoV-2 can infect people of any age, even if they are in good health and their immune system is working properly.

Only older people and people with previous medical conditions get complicated and die

Statistics managed by the WHO indicate that the highest rate of complications and mortality from COVID-19 occurs among the group of people older than 60 years or with underlying diseases such as diabetes, hypertension or cardiovascular diseases. However, this mortality is not limited exclusively to this group, since there is also a large percentage of those infected with ages between 20 and 59 years.

Healthy children and youth are less susceptible to COVID-19 disease

Although statistics of reported cases worldwide indicate a lower incidence of the disease among children from 0 to 10 years, this does not imply that they are less vulnerable to infection or may develop complications.

The possibility of contagion has been found to be equal to all ages, whether or not there are previous medical conditions. In many countries, children with respiratory symptoms are not tested, which may affect COVID-19 statistics in that group.

There are currently several studies underway to identify whether or not there is some type of natural mechanism that is more resistant to young organisms in adults and older adults against cell invasion by SARS-CoV-2.

Difference between protective inflammatory and hyperinflammatory response

As an initial reaction to an infection or injury, the body activates an inflammatory immune mechanism that helps repel pathogens and repair tissues.

In the case of those infected with COVID-19 who develop mild or moderate symptoms, some type of inflammation is present in the lung tissues, which are the first to be attacked by the SARS-CoV-2 coronavirus. This inflammation aims to protect the body against the progression of this infection.

However, in many cases, COVID-19 causes a hyperinflammatory response that practically floods the lungs with fluid, which in turn leads to organ failure and death.

This reaction is similar to what happens in patients with advanced autoimmune diseases or who suffer serious infections.

COVID-19 patients can go from having symptoms similar to a normal viral picture to suffering an extreme inflammatory process in a very short period of time. In addition to the lungs, other organs such as the heart are also affected by this hyperinflammatory process.

The use of some medications to treat rheumatoid arthritis, such as tocilizumab, has given good results in seriously ill patients who were initiating a severe inflammatory process.

In most cases, having to intubate them after lung function normalized with the use of this drug was avoided.

Cytokine storm and hemophagocytic lymphohistiocytosis

COVID-19 provokes an exaggerated and uncontrolled immune response in severe patients called "cytokine storm". In its fight against the infectious agent, the immune system destroys the cells of the pulmonary epithelium, causing the lungs to become inflamed and fill with fluid and phlegm. This in turn causes respiratory failure or sepsis that can be fatal.

The cytokine storm is believed to have been responsible for many deaths in the 1918 Spanish Flu pandemics and SARS in 2003. The autopsy of some who died of COVID-19 showed that they suffered from a hyperinflammatory syndrome known as secondary haemophagocytic lymphohistiocytosis (SHLH). SLHS can appear in adults affected by viral infections, who suffer from fulminant hypercytokinemia, as well as failure of several organs at once, including the lungs, with fatal results.

Renin axis angiotensin aldosterone: RCT vs ECAII

The renin angiotensin aldosterone axis (RAAS) is a cascade of vasoactive peptides that participate in key physiological processes.

SARS-CoV-2 enters lung epithelial cells using the angiotensin-converting enzyme 2 (ECAII) as a receptor.

The ECAII enzyme physiologically participates in the function of RAAS but also functions as a receptor for the coronavirus. In fact, it is considered that the lack of ECAII receptors in healthy children and youth could explain why COVID-19 does not seem to affect them as much as it does the older age groups.

Some experts have questioned the advisability of continuing to administer hypertensive drugs, which act as inhibitors of the RAAS axis, to patients with COVID-19.

The opinion is that it is not clear how RAAS blockers affect ECAII levels and activity and therefore, instead of improving the patient's resistance to infection, the opposite effect could be achieved.

However, other authors consider that removing these blockers could endanger the health of patients with COVID-19 with previous complications such as heart failure, myocardial infarction and other chronic heart diseases.

Does it help to stop treatments for hypertension, diabetes and rheumatoid arthritis?

In patients with diabetes and hypertension COVID-19 can cause serious imbalances that are life-threatening, so it is not advisable to alter or suspend treatment to control these conditions.

For autoimmune diseases like rheumatoid arthritis and others that require corticosteroid treatments, doctors have found that some medications interrupt the body's inflammatory response to COVID-19 infection.

This can be useful in severe cases where dangerous inflammation of the lung tissues is present. In any case, stopping these medications will depend on the decision of the treating doctor exclusively.

Loss of smell and taste as an initial symptom

COVID-19 patients worldwide have reported almost total loss of smell and taste at the onset of illness, even before the most typical symptoms such as fever, dry cough, tiredness, and difficulty breathing appeared.

A study published in April 2020 in California, United States, confirmed that the loss of these senses was common in 80% of those affected by COVID-19. However, it was also found that patients regained taste and smell 2 to 4 weeks after infection.

Useful warning signs for isolated minor patients in your home to avoid dying at home

Patients with mild conditions who are quarantined at home only require rest, hydration, and good nutrition during the 2-4 week period that may take time for the coronavirus infection to subside.

However, if at any time symptoms such as vertigo, blue tones in the nails and lips, chest pain and shortness of breath appear, medical help should be sought immediately as these are signs of possible complications in the lungs and circulatory system.

Differences in pathogenesis, clinical and treatment between the phases of COVID-19

COVID-19 has some important differences from other coronavirus diseases such as SARS and MERS. The first is its very high contagion rate, which contrasts with its low mortality rate.

COVID-19 fatality is between 1.5 and 2.4% of cases, compared to SARS and MERS, which had fatal rates of 11 and 30 percent, respectively. Although the initial symptoms are similar (fever, dry cough, and shortness of breath), COVID-19 also includes loss of smell and taste, stomach upset, and vertigo.

Because the majority of COVID-19 patients have mild symptoms, they can rest at home, while in SARS and MERS all those affected had severe symptoms that warranted immediate hospitalization.

All pneumonias require X-rays, ultrasounds and tomography

The protocol for the care of patients with COVID-19 indicates that they should have a chest x-ray and a blood oxygen analysis as a way of evaluating whether they are at risk of respiratory complications, such as pneumonia.

Patients with pneumonia should undergo radiological and ultrasound studies to monitor COVID-19 damage to the lungs.

These studies also allow us to know how much lung surface has been affected by the accumulation of phlegm and inflammation of the pulmonary epithelium, as well as to determine the level of evolution and response to the applied treatments.

Difference between RT-PCR and rapid diagnostic tests for SARS-CoV2

The RT-PCR or "Polymerase Chain Reaction" test is used to diagnose the presence of infection by detecting a fragment of the genetic material of the causative pathogen, be it a virus or a bacterium.

In the case of COVID-19, the RT-PCR test is applied to samples taken from the patient's upper respiratory tract. The objective is to detect a genetic fragment of SARS-CoV-2, that is, an RNA molecule corresponding to this coronavirus.

The RT-PCR test requires several hours to show the result, but it has a high hit rate.

For its part, rapid diagnostic tests do not detect the presence of the coronavirus causing COVID-19, but instead detect the antibodies produced by the organism infected with SARS-CoV-2, through a reactive and visual method based in colors, similar to pregnancy tests. Only one blood sample needs to be analyzed. The result is obtained in just 15 minutes.

Procalcitonin as a marker of bacterial infection

Procalcitonin is a serum polypeptide present in low amounts in the blood plasma, which increases its level considerably shortly after a severe systemic bacterial infection such as meningitis, septic shock or sepsis occurs.

In cases of localized bacterial infections such as pyelonephritis and pneumonia, its level increases moderately, while it remains stable in cases of viral infection or bacterial colonization.

For this reason, procalcitonin (PCT) is currently considered the best marker for the presence of bacterial infections, exceeding in effectiveness the count of leukocytes, C-reactive protein or interleukins.

Difference between extrapulmonary symptoms and multi-organ failure

The presence of abdominal pain, diarrhea, and vomiting was reported by many patients with mild to moderate symptoms of COVID-19 during the initial phase of the disease.

A percentage of these did not develop other COVID-19 symptoms such as fever, cough, or respiratory distress, but they maintained abdominal problems throughout their convalescence.

In severe patients, the main non-lung related problems were kidney failure, liver failure, myocarditis, and neurological problems stemming from hypertension.

Severity or mortality predictors that allow taking advanced medical actions

Different case studies of COVID-19 in China and Europe conclude that there is a set of predictors of severity or mortality among infected patients that must be considered by medical teams when deciding on the treatment to apply. These include the age of the patient, the presence of underlying medical conditions or diseases, the appearance of secondary infections, and the appearance of elevated inflammatory indicators in blood tests.

Other predictors of severity or mortality are leukocytosis, elevation of alanine amino transferase (ALT) and lactate dehydrogenase (LDH), increase in prothrombin time, and elevation of procalcitonin, serum ferritin, or interleukin levels. patients with higher SOFA scores also developed serious or fatal complications.

When to use olsaltamivir and other antivirals?

Because COVID-19 is a self-limiting acute disease, many patients with mild to complicated symptoms are receiving antiviral treatments as a strategy to shorten the duration of symptoms and reduce their severity. This type of strategy has been used successfully in the past in diseases such as Ebola, Hepatitis B and Ce, HIV and SARS.

There are currently more than 30 antiviral drugs on trial to determine their effectiveness against COVID-19, but all researchers agree that they are more efficient if applied when the first symptoms appear.

Use of ivermectin or nitazoxanide

Ivermectin has been used successfully in the treatment of dengue, Zika and influenza viruses and has the advantage of having few side effects. A study by Australian researchers indicates that applied in cultures of infected cells, this drug considerably reduces the burden of SARS-CoV-2 coronavirus in just 24 hours. In addition, in 48 hours this charge disappears completely or propagation ceases.

However, no tests have been performed on humans infected with SARS-CoV-2 and the dose required to achieve a laboratory-like result is still unknown. For its part, there are proposals to use the antiparasitic nitazoxanide in mild cases of COVID-19. This drug has already been used with promising results in the treatment of hepatitis C.

Use of azithromycin, chloroquine, and hydroxychloroquine

Chloroquine is a medicine used in the treatment of malaria and autoimmune diseases such as lupus or rheumatoid arthritis, which seems to have an antiviral effect against SARS-CoV-2 as it alters the pH of cellular lysosomes, where the virus multiplies. It also has anti-inflammatory effects that reduce the chance of lung damage from the cytokine storm.

Hydroxychloroquine is a chloroquine-based drug but with some chemical differences. However, its use has not been approved by the WHO, although the US government approved it under a health emergency decree in late March 2020.

Both medications can cause side effects such as headache, loss of appetite, vomiting, and skin rashes, and combined with azithromycin can cause cardiac arrhythmias.

Usefulness of fresh plasma or immunoglobulins from recovered patients

Studies are currently being carried out to determine whether fresh blood plasma and immunoglobulins extracted from patients recovered from COVID-19 can be useful to increase the immune response of healthy patients or decrease symptoms in those infected. This builds on some previous experiences with Ebola, as well as fighting chickenpox.

Throughout the month of April, companies in the United States and Europe advance the collection of plasma from patients recovered from COVID-19, rich in antibodies. They hope to have the first immunoglobulin-based therapy against SARS-CoV-2 after July 2020.

Temporarily, USA authorized the transfusion of plasma from recovered patients to very serious patients, as an extreme measure to save their lives through overstimulation of their immune system.

Use of interferons, monoclonal antibodies and intravenous immunoglobulins

Interferons are being tested and applied in the treatment of COVID-19 as a way to quickly stimulate the body's ability to react to infections by viruses such as SARS-CoV-2. Monoclonal antibodies have been used for years in the treatment of cancer and recently came to light as an effective way to fight Ebola.

Italian scientists are studying how to obtain monoclonal antibodies specific for SARS-CoV-2, which will require a shorter time than the development of a vaccine. B cells from patients recovered from the disease are used for this.

For its part, intravenous immunoglobulins have been useful to fight infections in patients in septic shock or sepsis and now we are investigating how to use them to specifically attack SARS-CoV-2.

The United States authorized this research and is working with some European companies to produce convalescent plasma, rich in antibodies, taken from patients recovered from COVID-19.

Troponins, enzymes, endothelial damage, heart damage, and acute myocardial infarction

In older COVID-19 patients with underlying cardiovascular disease, these were found to show signs of increased damage to heart tissue that could lead to acute myocardial damage.

Cytokine storm caused by lung infection in many cases caused death from fulminant myocarditis. COVID-19 has also been found to cause increased tension in the tissues of the heart due to the drop in blood oxygen levels due to involvement of the lungs.

Priority of the protection of the personnel before a cardiorespiratory arrest

Health personnel outside the health center, such as ambulances and similar services, must be protected with individual protective suits before treating any suspected or confirmed COVID-19 patient who suffers from cardiorespiratory arrest (PCR).

All resuscitation procedures should be avoided if the personnel do not have the basic personal protective equipment on, such as a mask, goggles, gloves and a gown. The practice of checking the patient's breath or applying mouth-to-mouth breathing should be avoided at all times. Using a defibrillator can quickly resuscitate the patient and avoid applying chest compressions and mouth-to-mouth breathing. If this does not happen, you should limit yourself to applying chest compression only.

In hospital settings, healthcare personnel should use all COVID-19 contagion protection tools and provide orotracheal intubation as quickly as possible while performing chest compressions or applying a defibrillator.

Improve airway while unemployed: laryngeal masks and entotracheal intubation

Patients with COVID-19 who require respiratory support by PCR can infect healthcare personnel by receiving mouth-to-mouth respiration, tracheal intubation, tracheostomy, non-invasive ventilation, or bag-mask ventilation.

If a laryngeal mask is used, a filter must be applied to it to prevent the patient's respiratory droplets from escaping into the air. As soon as possible, respiratory aid with entotracheal intubation should be given, trying at all times to wear personal protection elements such as a mask, face shield, gloves and full gown.

In cardiac resuscitation: defibrillation, pronation cardiac massage technique, medication

The high contagion capacity of COVID-19 requires changing the methods used for resuscitation of patients in cardiorespiratory arrest, in order to protect healthcare personnel.

Resuscitation procedures performed outside the hospital setting should be based as much as possible on the use of automatic external defibrillators (AEDs), rather than traditional cardiac massage or manual compression techniques. This increases the possibility of the patient reacting and avoiding having to maintain more physical contact.

Among the procedures adopted to aid the breathing of patients with acute respiratory failure, the prone position stands out. This relieves the pressure on the lungs and helps to increase the level of oxygen in the blood, reducing the need to intubate the patient.

In many cases of severe COVID-19 patients who suffered respiratory arrest while in pronation, a technique similar to that used for resuscitation of nursing infants has been applied.

In this case, a hard surface is placed under the patient's chest while applying rapid pressure or a series of blows to his back, to achieve chest compression that helps the heart to come out of the arrhythmia or regain its heartbeat.

Medication from a COVID-19 patient who has undergone cardiopulmonary resuscitation is a sensitive issue. Some patients are being experimentally treated with chloroquine and the like have suffered cardiac arrhythmias, so if they undergo a PCR, it is not recommended to continue applying this medication to avoid further damage.

Physicians have so far agreed on the importance of COVID-19 patients with heart problems continuing to receive medications for these conditions to reduce the chance of increasing damage to the heart and vessels.

Before cardiac damage: echocardiogram, interventional coronary angiography, and thrombolysis

One of the lessons learned from the COVID-19 pandemic is that patients with previous underlying conditions such as hypertension or acute coronary syndrome (ACS) are at high risk for serious complications and even death.

This has forced health professionals to rethink the protocols established for the care of coronary patients affected by COVID-19.

A large percentage of severe cases of this disease are related to patients with heart disease, who usually have an elevation of troponins of between 8 to 12%.

They also face the risk of developing myocarditis.

For this reason, health services should prioritize the use of non-invasive procedures when clinically evaluating a patient with risk of ACS or heart damage who is affected by COVID-19.

Care should be taken when deciding to perform interventional coronary angiography or any invasive procedure, and experts recommend performing it only if high-risk ACS or recurrence of ischemia is suspected even when treatment is applied.

However, the most important and recommended thing is to do this type of procedure only if the patient affected by COVID-19 has a good prognosis in his infectious picture.

Helps the immunomodulatory effect of statins: propolis, homeopathic drops and levamisole

A proposed strategy in the fight against COVID-19 is to apply anti-inflammatory drugs together with stimulants of the immune system, or immunostimulators. The anthelmintic drug Levamisole has been considered for this for its immunomodulatory properties, which help to increase the number of lymphocytes and strengthen the body's defense capacity.

It can also bind to the papain-like protease (PL-pro) present on the surface of SARS-CoV-2 and reduce its ability to infect human cells. There are also proposals to use natural products such as propolis, produced by bees, which is high in iron, aluminum, and antiseptic substances.

Added to this is the use of herbal homeopathic drops that have been shown for centuries to have properties to help the immune system. However, these therapies are considered to be alternatives and do not directly attack the COVID-19 infection but only help the body to have greater resistance to diseases in general.

Increase defenses: vitamin D, B-complex serums and vitamin C overdose

Although no direct relationship has been found between vitamin intake and protection against SARS-CoV-2 infection, some studies suggest that high-dose vitamin D therapy may help decrease the rate of infection in adults. young and old.

This is based on studies done on the incidence of cases in countries with less or more exposure to sunlight, which found that tropical countries tend to show a much lower rate of contagion than countries in the northern hemisphere.

The consumption of vitamin C or B complex does not seem to have a greater incidence in the treatment of COVID-19, although its consumption is recommended to maintain a healthy immune system.

Effective vaccines may be available in less than 2 years

Experts from all over the world assure that SARS-CoV-2 cannot be totally eradicated, so there is an urgent need to create a vaccine to protect the population. In January 2020, the genome of the SARS-CoV-2 coronavirus, responsible for COVID-19, was released, and the first experiments to create a vaccine against this disease were started.

More than 25 companies and laboratories around the world are working on the development of an effective vaccine against COVID-19, with the support of governments and public and private institutions. It is estimated that the first vaccine could be ready in about 18 months, that is, for the second half of 2020.

Thanks to international collaboration, this time frame is much less than what is normally required in a new vaccine, which may require up to 10 years of research and testing.

Does it affect pregnancy, childbirth and the newborn?

Studies done in Wuhan, China, pregnant women infected with COVID-19 found no signs of transmission of the virus from mother to fetus during pregnancy. This implies that the formation of the fetus is not affected by SARS-CoV-2, nor is there a direct risk that the newborn will contract the infection via the uterine route. However, if there were deaths of pregnant women who, before contracting COVID-

19, had already developed complications of pregnancy such as gestational diabetes or high blood pressure.

Cases of contagion have also been recorded in infants under the age of 1 year, which in some cases developed severe symptoms. In pregnant women with mild or asymptomatic symptoms, delivery could be carried out normally, but those with respiratory complications had to undergo caesarean sections to avoid risks to the life of the mother and child.

Will infected children have psychomotor and mental development problems?

So far it is unknown if COVID-19 leaves long-term consequences on the intellectual and psychomotor development of infected children, although there are several studies underway on this topic.

COVID-19 is known to have some neurological complications, such as loss of taste and smell, which usually recover 2 to 4 weeks after infection ends. Up to 36% of those infected show this loss of taste and smell or another neurological manifestation such as vertigo and headache. In severe cases, involuntary loss of breath control has been reported.

Are recovered patients immune to SARS-CoV-2?

Hospitals in China and South Korea that cared for patients with COVID-19 at the peak of the pandemic reported cases of reinfection in patients who had been discharged.

There are currently several studies underway that seem to indicate that the human body does not develop full immunity against COVID-19, so recovered patients have been recommended to follow sanitary hygiene measures and prevent infection, especially if they maintain contact with sick people in their homes.

Can recovered patients stop isolation and wearing masks?

Due to the possibility that recovered patients may be reinfected with COVID-19, the WHO has recommended that those discharged continue to apply preventive measures against contagion. This includes wearing masks and gloves when going outside and maintaining the recommended social distance from the rest of the population.

In addition, it has been found that some patients with mild symptoms of COVID-19 continued to be contagious for up to 8 days after symptoms ceased. For this reason, recovered patients are advised to maintain social isolation and precautionary measures for at least an additional 14 days, especially if they share a home with uninfected people.

Leaves functional sequelae or pulmonary fibrosis in recovered patients

Studies done to the lungs of serious or deceased patients by COVID-19 show serious damage to the pulmonary vessels, bronchi and bronchioles as a result of the disease. COVID-19 first destroys the hair cells of the pulmonary epithelium, responsible for "sweeping" bacteria, dust, and dead cells from the lungs. This causes a serious accumulation of phlegm and liquid in them.

In severe and fatal cases, it was found that patients lost up to 70% of their respiratory capacity due to the formation of plaques called "ground glass opacity" and inflammation of the lung epithelial tissue.

It has also been determined that the longer the lung inflammation or pneumonia lasts, the greater the permanent damage to the lung tissues.

109. The world after COVID-19

Among all the pandemics recorded in the Modern Age, the disease COVID-19 caused by the SARS-CoV-2 coronavirus is undoubtedly the one that has marked the most profound and extensive social structures on the planet. The degree of infection achieved by COVID-19 was notorious. In April 2020, it had already reached 2.4 million people in 225 countries and territories and caused 164,000 deaths.

The reaction of governments and population to the pandemic caused a profound change in the functioning of society and the economy, affecting more than 4.5 billion people. For the first time since the medieval black plague, entire countries ordered the total quarantine of their large cities, the cessation of non-essential commercial or industrial activities and the application of strict sanitary measures for those who had to go out to buy food, food or work.

Most regrettable was the massive death of older adults in countries like Italy and Spain, many of them in nursing homes where they hoped to calmly reach the end of their lives. Medical personnel were badly hit by COVID-19, with thousands of sick or dead doctors and nurses worldwide in just a few months.

However, the COVID-19 pandemic will also leave positive changes for society in the long term. For the first time since World War II, the health deficiencies of developed countries, which until then boasted of being organized and efficient in terms of health, were revealed.

This will force an in-depth review of their health systems, as well as the functioning of public and private organizations that must ensure the research and development of cures against diseases.

All countries alike should design response plans for future events of this magnitude, as well as improve the provision of equipment and medicines in hospitals and protect medical personnel, the first battlefront in the fight to save lives from diseases and disasters caused by man and nature.

For the first time, criticisms have been leveled at the functioning of untouchable institutions, such as the World Health Organization (WHO) and the Centers for Disease Control, and calls for greater democracy in decision-making within them. Another change will be seen in the behavior of the population, who will now understand the importance of taking care of hygiene standards to prevent the transmission of diseases.

The long social isolation applied in the big cities of the world will also change the way of interaction between people. Far from returning to the large crowds that have characterized urban centers, many people will now be more careful at the risk of getting sick. This will help reduce the incidence of communicable diseases like influenza, which claims thousands of victims each year around the world and which no one is talking about at the moment.

Nature will also benefit from this situation. The closure of large cities allowed a reduction in air pollution levels to be seen in a few days.

In India, for example, in just 15 days of quarantine the air was so cleaned that the Everest mountain range was visible from hundreds of kilometers away for the first time in more than 60 years. In Venice, Italy, fish were seen for the first time swimming in the calm waters of their canals, clean of sediment for the first time in decades. Dolphins and whales were seen daily in the vicinity of Italian and French ports, while wild animals such as goats and wild boars roamed the streets of English and Spanish cities with complete tranquility. This pause in human activity served for everyone to understand the beauty of Nature and the importance of protecting the flora and fauna that we still have.

In any case, the most important thing is that human life will be valued more, since this pandemic touched thousands of families who suffered the illness and death of their grandparents, parents, children and siblings. In a few months, the entire world will have overcome this pandemic and the lessons learned at the scientific, social and economic levels will allow Humanity to prepare so that such a situation does not recur, or reduce its effect if it occurs.

Finally, it remains to say that this publication has no other purpose than to serve as a guide on the current status of the COVID-19 pandemic and what is known about this disease at this time. Without a doubt, Humanity will emerge wiser from this situation and it only remains to hope that this lesson will serve to build a better future for all.

Epilogue

Final letter to my readers:

This is a battle that we all win.

This manual is designed to help you all better understand the new coronavirus, its effects and its consequences.

As it is a new and emerging situation, it is possible that much of the information included in this guide will be updated later, according to the evolution of the pandemic and the progress of investigations.

The urgency of the moment, and the need to disseminate current techniques to prevent and control the virus as quickly as possible, make the publication of this work necessary and indispensable.

Until a COVID-19 vaccine is available, the best way to deal with it is through collaboration, care, and shared experience. The more we know about the new coronavirus, the easier it will be to stop it and the less damage it will cause.

This is a battle that is only just beginning. There is still a lot to learn about COVID-19 and we still have a long way to go to beat it. However, I am convinced that we will, as we have done so many other times against even more deadly diseases.

This pandemic is a global problem that all humanity faces. The virus knows no borders and threatens all of us equally, without distinction of nationality, race, religion or social position.

We live in a unique moment, of uncertainty, panic, fear and anxiety, which forces us to reinvent ourselves. Whatever the outcome of this story, we will no longer be the same.

However, like any crisis, it is also an opportunity, an opportunity to be better, to put aside individualism and be more supportive. Not to seek to save ourselves alone and at any cost, and to lend a hand to the other. This moment is to forget the "*I conception*" and remember the "*idea of we*".

As much as the coronavirus forces us to isolation and physical distance, today we have to be more united than ever.

May this moment help us to get closer to our family and friends. May it help us strengthen communication with our children. This experience teaches us to protect our elderly and that we learn to take care of the health of our body and our planet.

In this sense, I hope that this manual will provide valuable information to the population in general and to health personnel in particular, and will serve to raise awareness of the importance of following preventive measures to prevent its transmission.

In the opinion of this author, it is feasible that the crisis will reach an acceptable control in October of this year, which will allow a return to normality in work, student and social activities in general. Although, according to the perspectives, and in the absence of specific vaccines and treatments, people will continue to get sick until 2022.

Everything will end by exhaustion of susceptible cases. This virus will exceed the possibilities of medical attention in all latitudes. Without a doubt, the world is and will be another, after the pandemic by COVID-19.

Before concluding, I want to leave my appreciation and admiration to all the colleagues who day by day risk their own lives to save those of others.

These heroes, many of them anonymous, are making a great effort to defeat this new threat. Together we make the impossible possible.

I leave you a hug full of hope.

Doctor Mario Vega Carbo

Endocrinologist

Content

The author...2

Volume 1 5

Introduction to Volume 1 6

Part I. Defenses, airways and viruses 12

   1. Types of Immunity. Examples 13

   2. Humoral and cellular immunity 15

   3. Active and passive immunity 16

   4. Defense against biological agents 17

   5. Anatomy of the airways 18

   6. Barriers, mucosa and respiratory epithelium.......19

   7. Acute respiratory infections 21

   8. Most common respiratory viruses......................22

   9. Bacterial over-infections 24

   10. Upper and lower respiratory complications 25

Part II Virology, Coronavirus and COVID-19 27

   11. Types and characteristics of non-respiratory viruses........28

   12. Flu and viruses more aggressive to the respiratory tree....30

   13. Coronavirus: types, their shape and structure 32

   14. Classification of coronaviruses 33

   15. Animal-borne coronaviruses 34

   16. Resistance in different environments 36

17. Differences between COVID-19 and previous coronaviruses..38

18. Virulence of SARS-CoV-2....................................38

19. Immunity to COVID-19 39

Part III. Risks and transmission between humans 42

20. Epidemiological characteristics.........................43

21. Most common transmission routes.....................45

22. Transmission by air drops 48

23. Transmission by indirect contact.......................49

24. Risks for closer contacts...................................51

25. Medical observation of contacts for 14 days....................52

26. Cutting the transmission chain 53

27. Risk groups more susceptible to contagion......................55

Part IV Cases, clinic and possible complications 57

28. Subclinical cases 58

29. Suspicious cases 59

30. Confirmed cases 60

31. Most common symptoms of the disease 60

32. Clinical signs to look for 61

33. Important laboratory tests................................62

34. X-rays and chest tomography............................66

35. Mild complications..68

36. Serious complications 69

37. Other complications 70

Part V. Community-acquired pneumonia..........................72

38. Concepts 73

39. Difference with nosocomial pneumonia 73

40. Diagnostic criteria 75

41. Causal pathogenic bacteria..................................76

42. Risk factors and prevention................................77

43. Viral pneumonia...79

44. Pneumonia due to COVID-19 80

45. Differences with other pneumonias...................81

46. Acute respiratory distress syndrome 82

47. Respiratory sepsis and septic shock 84

48. Complicaciones extra respiratorias 85

49. Multiple organ failure..85

50. Medical discharge for pneumonia 86

Part VI. High risk of mortality 88

51. Elderly people 89

52. Smokers...90

53. Alcoholism 91

54. Bronchial asthma...92

55. Cardiovascular diseases.....................................93

56. Chronic lung disease 94

57. Diabetes mellitus...95

58. Chronic kidney disease......................................96

59. Hypothyroidism...97

60. Adrenal insufficiency 99

61. Obesity 100

62. HIV / AIDS 101

63. Malignant tumors 102

64. Transplanted 103

65. Use of steroids 103

66. Immunosuppressed 105

67. Mentally ill and disabled 105

Part VII. Global and community epidemiology 107

68. Epidemics in the history of humanity 108

69. Previous coronavirus epidemics 108

70. Start, development and end of the pandemic 109

71. Possibilities of local endemics 111

72. Local, national and international measures 112

73. Quarantine and social isolation 114

74. Individual protection for the sick 115

75. Individual protection of your contacts 117

76. Protection of health personnel 118

77. Protection of security personnel 119

78. Declaration of cessation of quarantine 120

79. Declaration of cessation of transmission 121

80. Notifiable disease 122

Part VIII. Prevention of disease 123

81. Surveillance for symptom-free contacts 124

82. Caring for the patient with COVID-19 at home 125

83. Transfer of suspects or sick 126

84. Complicated hospitalization 127

85. Conjunctural hospitalization centers 127

86. Intensive care and assisted ventilation 129

87. General and immunological support measures 130

88. Antivirals, Antibiotics, and Steroids 131

89. Current and future vaccines.......................................134

90. Control of chronic patients..135

91. Vitamins and nutrition..136

92. Management of social and individual stress 137

93. Natural and traditional treatments 140

Part IX. Individual and collective protection 142

94. Weather care..143

95. Use and type of masks...144

96. Hand washing...146

97. Alcohol and antibacterial 147

98. Lifestyle, exercise and mental health 149

99. Ventilation of houses and rooms..................................151

100. Care in quarantine 151

101. Homes for the elderly and disabled...........................152

102. Markets and supermarkets.......................................153

103. Restaurants and dining rooms 154

104. Cinemas and theaters...155

105. Lifts and stairs 155

106. Public and private transportation..............................156

107. Flights and airports...157

108. Ports and cruises..158

109. Schools and universities 158

Part X. Summary of facts and clinical controversies 160

Volume 2 181

Novel-coronavirus Guide 182

Background and timeline of the pandemic.......................183

Part I. Defenses, airways and viruses 190

1. Types of immunity 192

2. Humoral and cellular immunity 193

3. Active and passive immunity...194

4. Defense against biological agents 195

5. Anatomy of the airways 196

6. Barriers, mucosa and respiratory epithelium...................197

7. Acute and respiratory infections 198

8. Most common respiratory viruses....................................200

9. Bacterial superinfections 201

10. Upper and lower respiratory complications 202

Part II Virology, Coronavirus and COVID-19 205

11. Types and characteristics of non-respiratory viruses 206

12. Flu and viruses more aggressive to the respiratory tree ..207

13. Coronavirus: types, their shape and structure 208

14. Classification of coronaviruses 210

15. Animal-borne coronaviruses 211

16. Resistance in different environments 212

17. Differences between COVID-19 and previous coronaviruses......213

18. Virulence of COVID-19......214

19. Immunity to COVID-19......216

Part III. Risk and transmission between humans......218

20. Epidemiological characteristics......220

21. Most common transmission routes......222

22. Transmission by air drops......223

23. Transmission by direct contact......224

24. Risks for closer contacts......225

25. Medical observation of contacts for 14 days......226

26. Cutting the transmission chain......227

27. Risk groups more susceptible to contagion......228

Part IV Cases, clinic and possible complications......230

28. Subclinical cases......231

29. Suspicious cases......232

30. Confirmed cases......233

31. Most common symptoms of the disease......234

32. Clinical signs to look for......236

33. Important laboratory tests......236

34. X-rays and chest tomography......238

35. Mild complications......239

36. Serious complications......241

37. Other complications......242

Part V. Community-acquired pneumonia......244

38. Concepts 246

39. Difference with nosocomial pneumonia 247

40. Diagnostic criteria 248

41. Causal pathogenic bacteria......................................249

42. Risk factors and prevention......................................250

43. Viral pneumonia...252

44. Pneumonia due to COVID-19 254

45. Differences with other pneumonias...........................255

46. Severe acute respiratory syndrome 256

47. Respiratory sepsis and septic shock 257

48. Extra respiratory complications 257

49. Multiple organ failure...258

50. Medical discharge for pneumonia..............................259

Part VI. High risk of mortality 261

51. Cardiovascular diseases..262

52. Elderly people 263

53. Smokers...264

54. Alcoholism 266

55. Bronchial asthma...266

56. Chronic lung disease 267

57. Diabetes mellitus 268

58. Obesity 270

59. Hypothyroidism...271

60. Suprarrenal insufficiency 272

61. Chronic kidney disease...274

62. HIV / AIDS 275

63. Trasplanted 277

64. Steroid use 278

65. Immunosuppressed...279

66. Mentally ill and disabled 280

Part VII. Global and community epidemiology 282

67. Epidemics in the history of humanity 283

68. Previous coronavirus epidemics......................................286

69. Start, development and end of the pandemic 288

70. Possibilities of local endemics 289

71. Local, national and international measures 290

72. Quarantine and social isolation 292

73. Individual protection for the sick 294

74. Individual protection of your contacts 296

75. Protection of the health professional..............................297

76. Protection of security personnel....................................299

77. Declaration of cessation of quarantine 300

78. Declaration of cessation of transmission........................302

79. Notifiable disease 302

Part VIII. Prevention of disease...304

80. Surveillance for symptom-free contacts.........................305

81. Caring for the patient with COVID-19 at home..............307

82. Transfer of suspects or sick..309

83. Complicated hospitalization 310

84. Short-term hospitalization centers..................................311

85. Intensive care and assisted ventilation 312

86. General and immunological support measures 314

87. Antivirals, antibiotics, and steroids 315

88. Current and future vaccines 317

89. Chronically ill control 318

90. Vitamins and nutrition 319

91. Management of social and individual stress 322

92. Natural and traditional treatments 324

Part IX. Individual and collective protection 326

93. Weather care 327

94. Use and type of masks 328

95. Hand washes 330

96. Alcohol and antibacterial 331

97. Lifestyle, exercise and mental health 332

98. Ventilation of houses and rooms 334

99. Homes for the elderly and disabled 335

100. Markets and supermarkets 337

101. Restaurants and dining rooms 338

102. Cinemas and theaters 339

103. Lifts and stairs 340

104. Public and private transportation 341

105. Flights and airports 342

106. Ports and cruises 344

107. Schools and Universities 346

Part X. Summary of facts and clinical controversies 348

108. Explanations on COVID-19 349

109. The world after COVID-19 376

Epilogue..380

Bibliographic references..395

The author...399

Other books 399

Social Network:..400

Synopsis..401

Bibliographic references

1.   "Cases of pneumonia in China's Wuhan could be due to a new type of virus: the WHO." YouTube. Retrieved on March 29, 2020.

2.   "New coronavirus - Thailand (ex-China)". WHO. January 14, 2020. Retrieved on March 29, 2020.

3.   "General Immunology Course". University of Granada. Microbiology Department. Retrieved on March 30, 2020.

4.   "Immune System: Cellular Immunity and Humoral Immunity". My Immune System. Retrieved on March 29, 2020.

5.   "Immunity against infectious agents". Page 99.J. Chabalgoity, M. Pereira, A. Rial (2008).

6.   "Important features and lessons of the 2019 coronavirus disease (COVID-19) outbreak in China". Femeba Foundation. Summary of the CDC report of the People's Republic of China on 72,314 cases. Retrieved April 1, 2020.

7.   "Modes of transmission of the virus causing COVID-19: implications for IPC precautionary recommendations". World Health Organization. Study published on March 27, 2020. Retrieved on April 2, 2020.

8.   "Severe Outcomes Among Patients with Coronavirus Disease 2019 (COVID-19)". CDC. March 2020.Retrieved on March 28, 2020.

9.   "Clinical evidence does not support corticosteroid treatment for 2019-nCoV lung injury". The Lancet.Russell CD, Millar JE, Baillie JK. February 7, 2020

10.   "Treatment for COVID-19 for you and the house." Mayo Clinic. Retrieved April 10, 2020.

11.   "Nonspecific (Heterologous) Protection of Neonatal BCG Vaccination Against Hospitalization Due to Respiratory Infection and Sepsis". María José de Castro, Jacobo Pardo-Seco and Federico Martinón-Torres. U.S. National Library or Medicine. Published June 1, 2015.

12.   "Pneumonia cases in China's Wuhan could be due to new type of virus: WHO". YouTube. Retrieved on March 29, 2020.

13.   "Novel Coronavirus - Thailand (ex-China)". WHO. January 14, 2020. Retrieved on March 29, 2020.

14.   "General Immunology Course". University of Granada. Microbiology Department. Retrieved on March 30, 2020.

15.   "Immune System: Cellular Immunity and Humoral Immunity". My Immune System. Retrieved on March 29, 2020.

16.   "Immunity against infectious agents". Page 99.J. Chabalgoity, M. Pereira, A. Rial (2008).

17.   "Important features and lessons of the 2019 coronavirus disease (COVID-19) outbreak in China". Femeba Foundation. Summary of the CDC report of the People's Republic of China on 72,314 cases. Retrieved April 1, 2020.

18.   "Modes of transmission of viruses causing COVID-19: implications   for   IPC   precaution   recommendations".

WorldHealthOrganization. Study published on March 27, 2020. Retrieved on April 2, 2020.

19.   "Severe Outcomes Among Patients with Coronavirus Disease 2019 (COVID-19)". CDC. March 2020. Retrieved on March 28, 2020.

20.   "Clinical evidence does not support corticosteroid treatment for 2019-nCoV lung injury". The Lancet. Russell CD, Millar JE, Baillie JK. February 7, 2020

21.   "Treatment for COVID-19 for you and the house". Mayo Clinic. Retrieved April 10, 2020.

22.   "Nonspecific (Heterologous) Protection of Neonatal BCG Vaccination Against Hospitalization Due to Respiratory Infection and Sepsis". María José de Castro, Jacobo Pardo-Seco and Federico Martinón-Torres. U.S. National Library or Medicine. Posted on June 1, 2015.

The author

Mario Vega Carbó

Physician- Endocrinologist

- Cuban doctor graduated in 1994.
- Specialist in Endocrinology and Family Medicine.
- Master in Longevity and Ultrasound.
- Professor of medical pathophysiology.
- Lover of doing good, family and nature.

Other books

1. A bet on natural endocrinology.

2. Answering 1,500 questions about: Hormones, metabolism and nutrition.

3. Where hormone reigns... fiction based on clinical cases.

4. S.O.S Hormonal toxics.

5. Reveling myths: Metabolism, Endocrinology and Reproduction.

6. Hormones, glands and endocrine diseases. Its story.

7. Coffee, tobacco and alcohol: Metabolic and hormonal disorders.

8. Endocrine alerts.

9. Novel coronavirus: guide.

Social Network:

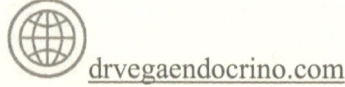 drvegaendocrino.com

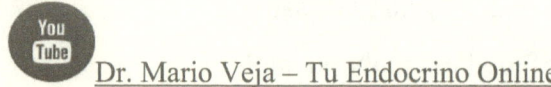 Dr. Mario Veja – Tu Endocrino Online

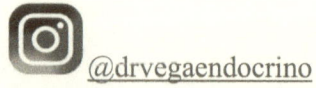 @drvegaendocrino

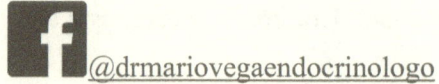 @drmariovegaendocrinologo

Synopsis

We live in a time that will be marked in history. Until a few months ago, hardly anyone had heard about the novel-coronavirus, and today its impacts plunged the world into an unprecedented global and social crisis.

As there is no concrete cure so far, the best way to deal with it is through knowledge, research and the dissemination of proven techniques to control and prevent it.

In this framework, Dr. Mario Vega Carbó presents a new book in which he fully explores the world of viral diseases.

In this book, he analyzes the history and characteristics of the new coronavirus, the way it is transmitted, its most common symptoms and the complications it generates in the human body.

It also delves into the groups at highest risk, the preventive and protective measures that should be taken, and the types of treatments available.

Due to the times, it is an essential reading manual for everyone.

www.ingramcontent.com/pod-product-compliance
Lightning Source LLC
Chambersburg PA
CBHW030605220526
45463CB00004B/1176